My Friendship with Yoga

Krishna *uvacha* (Lord Krishna says),

"Do thy work by being steadfast in yoga, abandoning attachment, free from selfish desires and be balanced in success or in failure. Yoga is evenness of mind."

{Bhagavad Gita – Chapter 2, Verse 48}

My Friendship with Yoga

Revathi Raj Iyer

Winspire
AN IMPRINT OF LIFI PUBLICATIONS
NEW DELHI

Published by:
WINSPIRE
An imprint of LiFi Publications Pvt. Ltd.
211, 2nd Floor, Gagandeep
12, Rajendra Place, New Delhi–110 008, India
Phone : (011) 2574 1000
E-mail : info@lifipublications.com
Web : www.lifipublications.com

ISBN 13: 978-93-86191-00-7 ISBN 10: 93-86191-00-8

First published in 2017

Cataloging in Publication Data—DK
[Courtesy: D.K. Agencies (P) Ltd. <docinfo@dkagencies.com>]

Iyer, Revathi Raj, author.
My friendship with yoga / Revathi Raj Iyer.
pages cm
ISBN 9789386191007

1. Yoga. 2. Hatha yoga. 3. Iyer, Revathi Raj. I. Title.

BL1238.52.I94 2017 DDC 294.5436 23

Printed in India by D.K. Fine Art Press (P) Ltd., Delhi–52

Raj, Shefali, and Patrick
(My strength and weakness)

My dear father & mother
for sincerely pursuing geriatric yoga

Dear Readers,

I dedicate this book to all those who are enthusiastic about yoga and wish to make it a part of their daily routine.

Enjoy yoga for healthy living and a happy feeling.

Namaste

Contents

Part 3. Daily Yoga Practice

Foreword

I am happy to write a brief Foreword to this book *My Friendship with Yoga*. The author of this book, Revathi Raj Iyer is an ardent follower of Yoga. She has studied the subject very well and also practises it in her daily life.

This book contains practical hints on Yoga so that everyone can practise Yoga. According to Worshipful Gurudev, Sri Swami Sivanandaji Maharaj, "Yoga is a complete life. Yoga is a science perfected by ancient seers of India. Yoga is the art of right living. Yoga is for all."

This book has been written in such simple and lucid language that everyone can easily understand and apply the principles in their day to day life.

The book contains several Yogic postures so that the student can easily follow and understand.

I wish many Yoga seekers should read it and derive immense benefit. I sincerely wish a wide circulation for this unique book.

May the benedictions of Worshipful Gurudev ever be upon all the readers!

Swami Vimalananda

President, The Divine Life Society

Sivanandashram, Post Shivanandnagar,
Rishikesh, Himalayas, Uttarakhand

24th September 2016

Acknowledgements

"When the doors close, a window opens," is an old adage which has been quite befitting in my search for a publisher. I would like to thank LiFi Publications Pvt Ltd for stepping in and opening that window for me. My heartfelt appreciation to the entire team of LiFi without whose acceptance, support and guidance this book would have been hibernating in my electronic folder. Bravo to the graphic artist for painstakingly fine tuning the illustrations several times over, until perfection.

My first yoga teacher Mr Syamala Prasad, deputed by the Indian Embassy to Fiji Islands, who introduced me to the rhythm of yoga and all my instructors at Flow Hot Yoga, Christchurch, New Zealand, who unknown to themselves, inspired me into deepening my yoga practice. Their Western twist made the sessions very intense, interesting and fun. Thank you all!

My gratitude and respect to Shri Swami Vimalanandaji for his kind Foreword.

Shri Prashant S. Iyengar, Ms Pinky Lilani, Ms Nanny A. Van den Oever and Ms Victoria Pomeroy – I am touched by your kind words about my book. Thank You!

The stalwarts of yoga Yogacharya B.K.S Iyengar, Dr Geeta S. Iyengar and Ms Donna Farhi, whose words of wisdom have been quoted in this book.

Carole and amma – I owe it to these lovely ladies for inspiring me to write and Shefali for her thoughtful inputs.

My friends and Facebook buddies for spreading the buzz.

I would like to express my deepest gratitude to the inmates of Sivananda ashram at Rishikesh, for their kindness, love and inspiration and the divine Ultimate for helping me put my thoughts into words and all those who have contributed in making my wish of reaching out to my readers, a reality.

Author's Note

This book is a seeker's guide for yoga enthusiasts as well as those who have been practising yoga in their daily life. It is not a treatise but a mix of facts, opinions and anecdotes, coupled with tips and techniques that I have learnt along the way. It should be borne in mind that the asana (postures) described herein are by and large for those who have no serious and specific health issues or ailments. Yoga is certainly meant for everyone, but those with specific health concerns are advised to first consult their physician before attempting any of the asana (postures).

For beginners, I would urge that the asana (postures) be performed under a trained instructor in order to fully understand the rudiments and techniques and thereafter follow the instructions as set out in this book. It is good to seek, learn and practise, in that order.

Curiosity is a virtue and we are on a learning curve, so even as one teaches and shares yoga with students one may wish to compare notes with this book to understand a student's journey.

I have quoted a couple of verses from the *Bhagavad Gita* as this ancient epic brings out the nuances of 'Brahma Vidya' which means knowledge of the Divine and 'Yoga Saastra' which are the Scriptures on yoga, to develop a receptive, calm and open mind that wishes to learn and evolve. I believe that yoga is not about asana (posture) alone, but is a spiritual path towards exploring the divinity within us and becoming a better human being. Keeping this in mind, a chapter on a typical day at an ashram has been included for the benefit of the readers. Pranayama (breathing technique) is a vast topic by itself and hence beyond the scope of this book. However, the basic pranayama exercise has been explained in Part 3 under the daily yoga practice.

Please bear in mind that this basic tenet of yoga which I abide by is my own practice:

"Do not ever force yourself into a posture. Do not try to be perfect. Keep trying until the asana (posture) grows on you. This is the path of yoga that teaches you to be resilient and patient. Patience, practice and perseverance alone can unlock this ageless tradition of yoga."

Part 1 – Narrative

1

Introduction

"What is yoga?" I asked a friend of mine.

She looked at me with wide eyes as if I was asking her a trivial question and remarked, "Revathi, everybody knows that yoga is a connection between mind and body."

I smiled and said, "Not everybody."

II

"How long does it take to start feeling this oneness?"

"Have you started feeling it?" I prodded as I was aware that she regularly attended a yoga class.

This time she looked at me with a thoughtful expression probably because she sensed that I was trying to make a point. She was a bit more guarded in her response and said, "I am not too sure. It might take a few years, a lifetime or maybe even beyond."

I smiled and said, "Just as I had expected."

II

"Why do you do it?" I asked.

"Why are you quizzing me? Are you writing a book?" she asked, impishly.

I nodded and said, "Yes, indeed! I have started writing my journal on yoga and perhaps someday it might take the shape of a book."

My friend replied, "I love yoga. It makes me feel content, cheerful, energetic and also keeps me fit. Good luck with your book," she added and we parted ways.

II

Readers, the point I am trying to make is that yoga can be interpreted in different ways. It is a unique experience to each one of us. It could mean an exercise, meditation and relaxation to some, an awareness of self via conscious breathing techniques to a few others and a joyful experience to the rest or even a dance, as my teachers would often describe it.

No matter what, all of these lead to the ultimate bliss – 'Union with God'.

A majority of you may be well aware that Patanjali, the sage of yesteryears, crafted the map of yoga through the yoga sutras or aphorisms. Some scholars believe that Patanjali was more of an exponent than a creator of yoga. Nevertheless, his aphorisms have come to be regarded as the 'Bible of Yoga'. Over the years, this tradition was mastered by the yoga gurus. They learnt and practised the techniques based on the sutras (aphorisms) and thus developed this beautiful art of yoga and the path to spirituality which has spread worldwide and is now a boon to mankind.

Yogacharya B.K.S. Iyengar in his book, *Yoga Wisdom & Practice* (for health, happiness and a better world) has beautifully brought out the nuances of yoga. He says, "Man is a product of *vidya* (intellect), *buddhi* (intelligence), emotion, action and determined will. While the seat of the intellect is the head, seat of the emotion is the mind. Hands and feet are meant to be the limbs for action. If one has to be pure in action, love (lust-free emotional life) or in intellectual pursuits, the foundation is the path of yoga."

This is a fascinating anecdote about sage Patanjali which I would like to share with you all. *{Courtesy bksiyengar.com}* As per this ancient legend, one day Lord Vishnu was invited to watch the *Tandav Nrittya,* the energetic Nataraja dance, by the one and only one, Lord Shiva. Lord Vishnu was so enthralled by it that his body started vibrating to the movements of the dance. Adisesha, the King Cobra, also known as the Serpent God, on whom Lord Vishnu rested, found this too hard to bear. He struggled to remain stable and started getting breathless. Adisesha waited desperately for the dance to finish. He was glad when the dance ended as Lord Vishnu's body became normal and light and he regained his breath.

Adisesha became curious and asked Lord Vishnu the cause for the sudden change that he had experienced during and after the dance.

To this Lord Vishnu replied, "My dear Adisesha, I was much captivated in Lord Shiva's dance that my body felt the vibrations and started moving automatically. This may have caused my body to become heavy and given discomfort to you." He apologised with a smile.

Adisesha felt very embarrassed and kept quiet. But he could not help thinking about it. He was so torn between envy and adoration of Lord Shiva that he decided to learn the dance, so as to impress his Master Vishnu. But there was a dilemma. He had to be born as a human being in order to do so. Thus began his quest for a mother who had to be a devout yogini and blessed by the sages for her unwavering penance. After years of search he found these qualities in Gaunika.

One day, as Gaunika was praying to the Sun God, she felt a creeping sensation. She opened her eyes and saw a small snake moving in her palms. She was terrified and begged the Sun God to forgive her.

He immediately appeared before her and said, "Gaunika, you have not committed any sin. You have been blessed with a son." Saying this, he disappeared and a bewildered Gaunika stared with astonishment at the sight of the snake writhing in her palms. At once the snake, none other than Adisesha, took a human form and with humility knelt before her.

Gaunika silently thanked the Sun God and gracefully accepted this God given child. She named him Patanjali which literally means, 'fallen into the hands at the time of prayer'. This also explains the reason behind Patanjali being depicted as half-human and half-serpent. A beautiful carving of this portrayal can be seen at the Ramamani Iyengar Memorial Yoga Institute, Pune.

The origins of yoga are very strongly tied to sage Patanjali. His yoga sutras or aphorisms define the eight fold path of yoga which lays down the guiding principles of this tradition. These have been dealt with appropriately elsewhere in the book.

2

My Foray into Yoga

It was in the beginning of the year 2004, in Fiji Islands, that I made up my mind to learn yoga. Prior to that, aerobics and strength training were my main fitness modes. As much as I hate to admit it, I harboured a misconceived notion about yoga, believing that it was meant for flexible bodies. I later realised how wrong I was!

As I started to read books written by eminent personalities and about the experiences of those who had been practising yoga consistently for several years, I began to understand the true spirit of this tradition and was filled with curiosity to find out whether yoga would work for me. I was in pretty good shape, both in mind and body – a happy person with a positive bent of mind and a self-possessed personality. I was also at that emotional juncture of life where my only daughter would eventually leave home for her undergraduate studies. Most of the decisions that I had made, as regards my career or moving away from India all the way to a far-flung island in the South Pacific, were centred round my daughter. Perhaps this was also one of the triggers that steered me towards yoga as a part of me wanted to feel more fulfilled and continue to remain in a happy state of mind and adapt to the changes that life can surprise us all with.

Thus began my foray into yoga and, in retrospect, I feel delighted that I buried my misconception and sought to understand yoga and reap its benefits at the right stage in my life, instead of waiting until age caught up with me.

Our instructor Mr Syamala Prasad was a disciple of Yogacharya B.K.S. Iyengar, the veteran yoga guru. He was therefore well-trained in yoga which involves various postures and limb movements using props. He never failed to brief us all about Yogacharya B.K.S. Iyengar and his lifestyle and we listened in rapt attention. Without having had the opportunity to meet him, I became an admirer of Yogacharya B.K.S. Iyengar. The manner whereby he has effectively passed the rich yogic legacy to his children, grandchildren and all his students is highly commendable.

Although he has passed away, the wealth of knowledge that he has left behind for the generations of today and all times to come by, will remain rock solid and he will always be remembered as an epitome of loving, giving and sharing.

My first yoga class was in a laid back small town named Lautoka. I went with an open mind and absolutely not knowing what to expect. We were asked to get bedspreads, cushions or pillows, a yoga mat and a water bottle. It felt as if we were going for a sleep therapy session. I was filled with excitement and scepticism but deep down I knew that this beginning was going to stay with me forever.

As we took our positions, I scanned the class. It was a happy mix of varying age profiles: some were close to my daughter's age, some were closer to my age and the rest were older than me. Strangely, the older persons appeared more calm and composed as compared to their younger counterparts. This added to my comfort level and I felt instantly better. I was apprehensive that my body may have lost its suppleness over the years in spite of my fitness training but I was confident that yoga would resolve this in course of time.

My first class was a shocker, indeed! Our instructor Prasad

had a Zen like look as he sat quietly in front of us. It appeared to me that he was meditating and looking beyond us, for some reason that I could not fathom. We were a hotchpotch from diverse cultures and in different shapes and sizes waiting to bombard him with questions, in a fit of enthusiasm and anxiety. Several questions went unheard and a few unanswered. He was still silent. Gradually, we slowed down on the verbal exercise and the class became extremely quiet, after the initial cacophony.

He then broke the silence. "This is the basic principle. Please maintain total silence during practice, listen to my instructions and try to follow them as much as you can. I will clarify your doubts after the session concludes," he said. There was pin-drop silence for a few minutes. We were asked to lie down on our mat and relax completely.

Our first session began with savasana, the corpse pose.

Although it looked simple enough, this posture was difficult to sustain as we had to be still as if in a state of meditation.

"Let go of all thoughts, allow them to pass and consciously focus on yourself, by diverting all attention to your breath," echoed the voice of the instructor, soft yet firm.

I tried my level best to follow his instructions but my mind was playing tricks and kept straying. I suddenly remembered having read about people who felt the kundalini (dormant energy) rise slowly from the base of the spine up to their foreheads with a sudden flash of light as if they had seen God.

As I lay on the mat with my eyes closed, trying hard to locate this energy, I must have stiffened my face, for just then I heard the instructor say, "Relax your facial muscles, relax your eyes and nose and so on."

He took us through the relaxation process of each and every part of the body. It felt nice. "Are you all following your breath? Are you all breathing deeply in and out? I have to see those belly movements," he insisted in his firm tone. This made me realise that I had not been with my breath at all.

Focussing on the breath is the most important aspect of yoga practice. This was one of the first vital lessons I learnt that day.

I listened to his words intently and adjusted my breathing pattern. Just when I started my rhythmic breathing, the instructor said he could not hear us at all. He wanted to hear us breathe. I wondered in my mind's eye as to how one could breathe loudly without sighing.

"The technique is simple," he said, as if reading my thoughts.

"It is called '*ujjayi* breathing', which is deep inhalation and exhalation through the nose but with a heavy sound emanating in a subtle manner, to produce an oceanic breath."

"It may take a while to master this, but eventually it will get very comfortable and become an auto process," he said, by way of an explanation.

"This type of oceanic breaths coupled with belly breathing (similar to the way babies breathe – with every inhalation the belly raises and contracts with exhalation) and engaging the bandhas, the interior body locks, is the master key to an energised mind and body," he further added.

My mind raced and I tried not to think about this new term, 'bandhas' (interior body locks). Fortunately he did not stress on this.

"Breathing is the prana, the energy or life force that sustains us," he continued.

I listened carefully to his words and tried to follow his instructions. It was a fantastic feeling as we came out of savasana, the corpse pose. We stretched our bodies with arms over the head and simultaneously flexed our toes, inwards and outwards. The instructor then asked us to come to a standing position with a quick jump.

Thereafter began the popular surya namaskar, the sun salutation series. This is a warm up sequence that strengthens our muscles, tissues, nerve endings and meridians; in nutshell, a complete body workout. This series comprises twelve steps, each being a specific asana (posture) that has to be done methodically and at a medium pace with breath synchrony, to derive the maximum benefits.

As I started my first surya namaskar (sun salutation), I felt my body tingle with a fresh feel. We completed six rounds, by which time the body had started to warm up. I ran a mild sweat. The instructor gave us an option to stop there and relax for a few breaths in the corpse pose, as this was our first class. But those who wanted to continue were allowed to do so till the completion of nine rounds. I managed to complete all the nine rounds and quickly sunk into savasana, the corpse pose, with a sense of achievement and relief. I could hear my heart pounding fast and my breath was faster. I closed my eyes and relaxed completely. Slowly and steadily, my body regained its normal breathing pattern and my heart beat became even and slow. I melted in that heavenly state.

This is when I learnt my second lesson: to be present 'in' the moment with a mind free from all thoughts and disturbances.

It was a wake-up call to remind me that I needed to work on training my mind. I have dealt with this in the next chapter.

The class finished with a prayer to sage Patanjali to whom the origins of yoga are strongly tied. We all joined our hands in prayer to thank Patanjali for having bestowed upon us the wonderful art of yoga.

Yogena cittasya padena vacam
Malam sarirasya ca vaidyakena
Yopakarottam pravaram muninam
Patanjalim pranjaliranatosmi
Abahu purusarakaram
Sankha cakrasi dharinam
Sahasra sirasam svetam
Pranamami Patanjalim

"To the noblest of sages Patanjali,
who gave Yoga for serenity of mind,
Grammar for purity of speech,
Medicine for health of the body. I bow,
I prostrate before Patanjali,
whose upper body has a human form,
whose arms hold a conch and disc,
who is crowned by a thousand-headed cobra,
The incarnation of Adisesha, my salutations to thee!"

{Translation courtesy – Yogacharya B.K.S. Iyengar & Dr Geeta S. Iyengar}

The end of my first yoga lesson proved to be a marvellous start for many more lessons to come thereafter. My affair with yoga had taken full form and shape. I started my yoga journal that night with a promise to stay committed in my practice.

In this book, I have shared excerpts from my journal, at appropriate places for the benefit of the readers. Hope you enjoy reading this book as much as I enjoyed writing it.

3

Thoughts and Monkey Mind – How to Tame it?

Human beings are endowed with an enormous capacity to think and this is an activity that we engage in abundantly and untiringly, each and every day. Just as the monkeys jump and cling onto branches of trees to move from one place to another, to pick fruits or follow their mates; similarly our untrained mind jumps from one thought to another without much purpose. Even when our body gets tired we keep thinking, unable to chase those thoughts away. When our thoughts get the better of us and start assuming alarming proportions, they can be counterproductive and affect our mind as well as body.

Is it not incredible that our brain processes as many as approximately 70,000 thoughts in a span of 24 hours? These thoughts generate mixed reactions in our minds and we tend to reach out for solutions to hypothetical situations succumbing to these highly volatile thoughts. For some, these thoughts keep working overtime and for others it is much calmer depending on the individual temperament. Every thought is not meant to be translated into action although we cannot stop mulling over it.

This is where yoga practice can help us by keeping our thought process under control and calming the mind. During practice, it is urged that we must consciously try to freeze our thoughts by focussing on the breath. We have to take charge of the monkey mind before it takes charge of us and this is by no means an easy task. It is probably easier to tame animals than our mind.

How can we not think? How can we possibly still our mind? The mind can be silenced for a few seconds, but then thoughts resurface to taunt us.

Many of you may have had a similar experience. There is nothing wrong with this. Remember, thinking is a natural trait and therefore we must learn to control our thoughts by not letting it find a permanent spot in our mind. Otherwise, with constant chatter, concentration becomes very difficult in yoga practice.

Isn't yoga supposed to help in concentration? Many of you might have this question pop up in your mind. My answer to this is that yoga will definitely help in improving concentration and inculcate a sense of discipline. But this can be achieved only when we consciously learn and practise to train our mind.

'How do we train our mind?'

The answer to this is, *'Learn to let go of your thoughts.'*

This does not mean that we stop or alter the process of thinking. It means that we try to let go of our thoughts as it occurs, let them pass by, channelling our mind and bringing the attention back to our breath. This is the meditational aspect of yoga.

Mind training is by no means an easy proposition. It will come only with time, patience and oodles of conscious practice. We have to be relentless in our pursuit. In spite of that, there will be days when our mind will refuse to obey but we have to keep trying until we reach a near meditative state.

Meditation is therefore an inseparable part of yoga training.

- In savasana (corpse pose), as we lie still, we learn to meditate.

- As we begin to hold postures for a few minutes, we learn to meditate.
- By consciously trying to focus on our breath, we learn to meditate.
- Whilst practising pranayama (breathing technique), we learn to meditate.
- Whilst chanting prayers, we learn to meditate.

In this manner we can improve our concentration as we do the various asana (postures) and automatically focus on our breath and inner self.

I would like to share with my readers a few steps that help me in meditation, relaxation and pranayama (basic breathing exercises). I hope this works for you, as well.

a) Sit comfortably without slouching. Try to keep the spine erect without causing any strain to the back.

   You may take wall support and sit on a cushion to slightly prop up your sit bones in order to keep the spine straight. If sitting on ground level is not comfortable, sit on a chair/ bench but remember to keep your back straight. Use support if needed. It is important to be seated comfortably.

   Vajrasana (thunderbolt pose) or padmasana (lotus pose) or ardha padmasana (half-lotus pose) are the various postures that are commonly used for this purpose. Just sitting comfortably cross-legged (Burmese style) with a cushion to support your back should also be well.

b) Start with deep inhalation (belly to expand with this intake of air and fill the lungs with a liberal dose of oxygen). Pause and exhale vigorously through your mouth. Repeat thrice to feel centred and relaxed.

   This should be followed by deeply inhaling, pausing, and

then exhaling via the nostrils, in a rhythmic pace.

As you do this, start counting the breath cycles up to the count of ten. Repeat this cycle a few times.

c) Try a mantra 'Aaa Ooo Mmm' (OM) in the silence of your mind.

d) Try counting a string of beads.

e) You could think of your most loved deity, if you are religious minded.

f) A pet can also be your focus of concentration.

g) Imagine a place of scenic beauty, a tulip garden, a lake with ducks or your own infant and focus on that image until it fades.

The essence of meditation is to channelise all your thoughts and bring them on to one point to keep your mind from straying. Sometimes your mind will simply refuse to be tamed. During such times, I remind myself of what I learnt from my instructors:

"It is important to stop when our mind starts misbehaving. We must at all times refrain from pushing ourselves, be it the mind or body. This is against the principles of yoga and meditation because anything forced will be counterproductive and may result in agitation of the mind or cause bodily injury. Both are not desirable."

I understood that it was wise to not be overambitious, at the beginning stages of meditation. Therefore it is best to sit and focus for five minutes to start with. Even this can be difficult if it is the first time. When you start to sense an improvement, gradually increase the meditation time to ten, twenty and thirty minutes.

It also helps to use the same spot for this practice. Probably the energy that is generated in that space augurs well. With practice you will begin to feel your breath getting calm, even, deep and long. You will start enjoying this romance with your breath. Once you have embarked on your journey, continue and do not give up. As the wise have said, "When you do the dishes, just do the dishes, feel the water against your hands, enjoy the soap bubbles, and see the dishes getting clean and nice as you place them in the drain basket."

The above is just an example to help readers understand how therapeutic a simple 10 minutes of your time in a day of twenty-four hours can be.

When I started to learn meditation, I would count from one to ten; after a while I would stop counting and turn my focus on the mild sound of my breath. When my mind started wandering, I would begin counting again.

Just to avoid monotony, I would mentally transport myself to my favourite island, take the help of a memory and imagine that I am collecting sea shells with my daughter. In my mind, I would start counting sea shells. This is my Zen practice and it helps in training the mind to concentrate better. You have to experiment and find out what works best for you.

I repeat, "Practice and patience is the key." You will eventually learn to trust yourself and your instincts.

"We are shaped by our thoughts, we become what we think. When the mind is pure, joy follows like a shadow that never leaves."

– Buddha

4

Decondition Your Mind and Let Go

Since childhood, our mind is conditioned due to several factors such as the influence of our parents, teachers, family, friends and to a large extent our faith, culture and the society that we live in. Our mind is programmed to act in a set manner. Over the years, this conditioning deepens and reaches a stage when it becomes hard to come out of it. Conditioning could be about behaviour, likes, dislikes, having an opinion, the way we look at things around us and ourselves.

Observe a child. The innocence, the joy, the act of doing something or not wanting to do anything, comes straight from the heart, free of bondage. This is the true nature of an unconditioned mind, the 'non-judgmental nature'. As young ones, we were more accepting, giving and not judging a situation or a person. But as we grow up conditioning of our mind begins unknown to ourselves. Sometimes we tend to second guess everything, to the extent of getting paranoid.

We strive for happiness but don't know how to go about it. We worry about career, how to make a living, how to raise children and so on. The 'what ifs' and 'how to' syndrome takes its toll over us emotionally and by middle age, we feel overwhelmed and given another chance we may wish to change the past.

Aren't we all too familiar with the term 'midlife crisis'? Who is responsible for this? Whom can we blame but ourselves?

Ask yourself questions like:

'Have I gone too fast in life?'

'Have my decisions been rational?'

'Am I being too hard on myself?'

There are no right or wrong answers. These are merely pointers to ponder about.

It is alright if we had made some mistakes as long as we had made those choices consciously or with a reason. Mistakes are not deliberate. They are accidental or guided by a situation that existed at that point of time in our lives. There is always a reason behind it. But if we start mulling over past decisions and ponder as to how life would have been if we had not made that choice – Oh well! Too bad because life does not work that way and may not give us a second chance either. One has to learn to move on even if it involves making adjustments and tougher decisions. These are the challenges of life that each one of us has to deal with. Therefore we have to try and remove the clutter from our minds to make a fresh start. This is the stepping stone towards our effort to decondition our mind in order to feel centred.

Just as the physical aspects (asana or postures) in yoga open up our body, at a plenary level, the meditative aspects of yoga open up our mind. This will help us to attain a balance between mind and body. Every posture done with passion and a sense of being with it will also open up our mind. This process should not be rushed or timed. It is a slow process of letting go of the past and living in the moment and acknowledging the present, without being anxious about the future. I cannot agree more in that it is extremely challenging to live in the present and enjoy each and every moment. "Easier said than done," people say. However we should feel blessed that with the help of yoga we can achieve this frame of mind provided we keep at it. It then becomes a two-way street to reckon with.

Here is what I look up to in my yoga practice: "Past has unfolded so it is time to let go; future is something we have no control over and so let go of that as well. What is left then? It is the present. We should cherish this wholeheartedly because very soon this present moment is going to be a thing of the past."

Here is a famous quote that I would like to share with you all.

"If you are depressed you are living in the past. If you are anxious you are living in the future. But if you are content you are indeed living in the present."

I have asked myself a million times as to how to let go. When we try to let go of certain thoughts they keep coming back. It is really hard to erase thoughts from our mind. Unfortunately, there is no delete button in our biological system. But we have to train ourselves and master this art of being at peace with our inner self and being in the moment.

A friend of mine shared with me an advice she sought from a monk. He asked her to write down on a piece of paper the list of things that she wanted to let go of. Then he asked her to concentrate and mindfully shred the paper to bits and trash it. Try and see if this works for you.

I follow another similar technique. I note down in my diary of the situations, memories, negative thoughts and emotions that I want to let go of. When I pen it all down from my mental diary, I feel a big sense of relief. Then I try and push it away from my mind. It is like blowing a bubble in thin air after taking a deep breath. Initially the art of letting go is a very conscious effort, but eventually it will become an auto process and stay in cruise control. It could slip at times, but we need to bring it back in the right gear.

An ardent yoga practice not only cleanses your system but also purifies your mind. We should always remember to not tread beyond our normal endurance or resistance levels, both in mind and body. We have to acknowledge the fact that each day is not going to be the same for us. This knowledge itself is the beginning of opening up and stabilising our mind.

I came across this thought provoking story of a centipede and the jealous tortoise written by Jostein Gaarder in *Sophie's World*. The sad part was that the centipede becomes a victim of a devious mind game played by the tortoise. Unable to let go of the thought wickedly planted by the tortoise, the centipede never danced again.

To me, the moral of this anecdote was that we must not overthink or overanalyse and shackle the mind to our own detriment and mental peace.

Feel the breath and enjoy.

Let go, let go, let go…

"Yesterday is but a dream, tomorrow is only a vision. But today well lived makes every yesterday a dream of happiness and every tomorrow a vision of hope, look well therefore to this day."

– Kalidasa

5

Intention and Determination

The rudiment of yoga practice is to be mindful in whatever we do, to be present in the moment and be aware of oneself. This is not going to happen overnight but it has to be cultivated through conscious effort and practice. Many yoga teachers suggest that we concentrate on our breath in order to cultivate the practice of being mindful. My yoga teacher followed a unique style. She would urge us to silently talk to ourselves and say, "I know I am breathing in," as we inhale and "I know I am breathing out," as we exhale, so that the mind and body complement one another and do not go in different directions. I found this very useful especially at the initial stages of practice.

Mind, body, inclination and determination are the most vital ingredients for daily yoga practice; rest all will follow. Well! This is what I kept telling myself when my affair with yoga first began. In a way, this is something we have to constantly remind ourselves of because there will be days or weeks when we may feel lazy or lethargic. Our mind will say a firm 'No' to our body and we will skip yoga for a day. A day will become few days and then weeks and not before long, we would have stopped practising yoga for months.

This is not uncommon for many, whatever the reasons may be. Some may find it very hard to resume especially after a brief illness. I have also gone through similar phases and understood that the only way to get back into the rhythm of yoga is through sheer self-determination. It boils down to the fact as to how passionate one feels about yoga. Falling sick, feeling lazy, losing momentum are all part of life. To make yoga a way of life, one has to acknowledge these and try to come back to it. Also, it is necessary to make time in your calendar, follow a timetable and make a commitment to oneself. Then see the difference!

My yoga teacher would ask all of us to bring our *sankalpa* (intention) to the mat. Nothing and nobody should matter during yoga practice. This is the time that we owe to ourselves, to energise and be able to continue with our day's activities with enthusiasm.

Look at a child when is engaged in something, howsoever trivial it may be. The child is admirably focussed and nothing will distract his/her attention. This is the same inclination that I am emphasising. Our inclination should be wholehearted, undivided and unconditional. This will help bring our sankalpa (intention) to the mat and it will seep into our daily yoga practice.

As we practise the various asana (postures), the sankalpa (intention) should also be for each and every move that we do on the mat. Only then will we be able to understand and learn as to how the mind listens to the body and vice versa. The minute we are distracted we have to necessarily come back to being mindful about our practice. This is the path of yoga.

I found a sweet and simple way of practising this concept. By dedicating my yoga practice each day to somebody close to my heart – a family member, a friend or even the Almighty – I could harness my sankalpa (intention) and my practice became mindful. Furthermore, sankalpa (intention) also keeps changing as our practice deepens. It may also vary from one day to another. Today my resolve could be that I should get fit and improve my stamina. Another time it could be that I am asking for patience and tolerance, yet another day I am just being grateful and so on. This sort of exercise instils positivity and a sense of well-being.

Let me also remind you that all this will not happen overnight and please don't be put off if it takes longer to achieve the desired result, in spite of having the will and determination. Our body responds to mental stimuli in its own way.

Let me give you my own example as to how I felt as I was writing this chapter.

My sankalpa (intention) to write a book on yoga took shape only because I started acting on it with determination and joy. However, when I started writing this book, I was not sure if I was going to self-publish it or contact an agent. I did not worry if my manuscript would reach the corridors of a publisher. But my sankalpa (intention) was firm. I had made a promise to myself that I would finish writing this book. It was not easy to find a publisher but eventually it happened. My sankalpa (intention) did not let me give up. As this book enters the competitive arena, I have no idea if it will be received in large numbers. I might even end up being out of pocket in making my book visible to you all. But my sankalpa (intention) is still in place and I am sure that my message will get across just as I have envisaged.

This principle applies to whatever we do in our lives and therefore it is imperative that we bring our sankalpa (intention) to our mats to enhance our yoga practice.

A quote from the veteran Donna Farhi, a renowned author and internationally acclaimed yoga trainer, is worth a mention here:

"Without intention all these postures, these breathing practices, meditations and the like can become little more than ineffectual gestures. When animated by intention, however, the simplest movement, the briefest meditation, the contents of one breath cycle are made potent."

Truth be told, such words of wisdom from stalwarts also help us in laying down our intention to achieve positivity and balance in our mind which bears an impact on our actions and decisions that we have to make in our daily lives. It builds confidence in our choices and makes us enjoy life for all that it is worth. We all live once; why not make it a most memorable and beautiful journey?

Mind, body, yoga mat, water bottle and oodles of sankalpa (intention) are all that we need to have a healthy practice. This is the mantra that I firmly believe in and which keeps me going.

6

Meridians and Chakras

I do not claim to be an expert on the topic of meridians and chakras, as this is one of the most complicated and subtle aspects in yoga practice. Conceptually it might seem simple to understand but how to adapt it in yoga practice is the challenge. We have to rely on our own ability to understand the energy points to be able to mindfully direct our breath towards these points. This technique together with engaging our bandhas (interior body locks) which is dealt with in the next chapter forms an integral part of a healthy yoga practice. Keeping this in mind, it is my humble attempt to put this chapter on meridians and chakras, in proper perspective.

Right from childhood we are only taught to believe what we can actually see such as tangible objects with some shape or form. Objects that are invisible to us often become a subject of our own imagination, but they have a significant relevance in yoga practice. For instance, we cannot perceive cosmic energy; however, this energy can awaken our spirituality no matter how esoteric this may sound, as our body draws energy from the cosmic environment whilst we practice the various asana (postures).

What are these so-called meridians?

These are the energy routes in our bodies that fortifies our immune system, restores balance and stamina, and makes us feel good. These meridians ensure flow of prana, the life force energy. The major meridians that run in the inners of our body are the lungs, heart, stomach, pancreas, spleen, intestines, gall bladder, kidney and liver, in addition to numerous other governing vessel meridians.

Our body gives a wakeup call when this energy is depleting, making us feel tired and irritable with all the endless daily activities – chores, hobbies, catching up with friends, bonding with relatives, spending time with family, trying to fit in an exercise routine…the list is endless.

Energy blockages can also happen if we are overworked and fatigue has cast its ugly shadow on us. This is harmful and can affect our immune system. Sometimes excessive flow of energy can be counterproductive and it can make a person hyperactive. Therefore it is vital to have a harmony in the flow of energy for our overall well-being.

The various postures and breathing exercises help to clear energy blockages and allow a natural and smooth flow of prana (life force energy) in our body. The postures massage the meridians and the internal organs, enabling us to clear the blockages as we breathe in, by listening to our body. The asana (postures) ensure smooth and steady flow of prana, the life force energy, only if we learn to focus on our breath and synchronise our breathing pattern with the asana (postures) throughout our practice. Automatically our breath will reach the meridians and start re-energising them leaving us rejuvenated after a session.

In the Western world, yoga focusses on the aspects of meridians. This is partly because of the popularity of Chinese medicine and acupuncture of the Eastern world that have gained momentum in the West. On the other hand, the term chakras are more familiar and well-understood in India, owing to alternative healing remedies, such as healing by touch (reiki) and ayurveda treatments, all of which relate to our body chakras.

What are these chakras? Chakras are the energy nodes present in our body and, like meridians, relate to the human organs. Starting from the base of the spine, these chakras traverse upwards to the crown of the head. The root chakra (kundalini) is at the base of our spine, and then comes the sacrum plexus (just below the navel), the solar plexus (base of the rib cage), the heart, throat, eyebrows and the crown chakra.

The scientific study of these two vast subjects is beyond the scope of this book. However, it is widely believed that yoga postures kindle our chakras (energy nodes) and helps the flow of prana (life force energy) in the right direction as we consciously become aware of our breath.

7

Bandhas (Interior Body Locks)

This is an extremely significant aspect of yoga practice. Simply stated, bandhas are the body locks that can be controlled by voluntary action. When I first heard this term, I was fascinated and confused at the very idea of being able to internally lock our body.

Let me start with a simple analogy. When we park our vehicle, we automatically bring the gear to a neutral position and turn off the ignition to conserve the battery, isn't it? In the same way, engaging our bandhas (interior body locks) helps us to conserve and channel the flow of energy or prana within our system, leaving us refreshed and energised after yoga practice. It took me awhile to understand this technique and several attempts to get it right.

We should never forget that yoga is all about learning day after day, month after month and year after year.

Let me start with my own experience to help you understand how this works. When I started learning yoga, I was clueless about this term. Fortunately, our instructor was kind enough not to introduce such intricacies initially as he did not want to intimidate us so that we continue yoga practice for a long time, even though he may have made passing references to this term. Personally, I would have been very disturbed had I been asked to focus on bandhas (interior body locks) along with breath awareness.

I learnt about bandhas (interior body locks) much later after gaining some level of confidence in the basic asana (postures) and breathing pattern. This also made me realise that initially one has to learn and practice with awareness so as to understand how to hold onto the bandhas (interior body locks) consciously, until it becomes an auto process whereby one could harmonise bandhas (interior body locks) along with breath.

Even after almost more than ten years of yoga practice, I sometimes tend to miss engaging my bandhas (interior body locks) and have to consciously remind myself to do so.

There are three bandhas – *mula bandha* (root lock), *uddiyana bandha* (abdominal lock) and *jalandhara bandha* (throat lock).

Let us examine these.

Mula Bandha (Root lock) – I apologise for having to explain this in a rather crude manner. But this is how my teacher explained it to me. Verbal explanation seems less crude and hilarious than reading it in fine print.

Imagine you have to urinate and are in a lecture/seminar and feel hesitant to ask for permission to step out or on your way home the snarling traffic has come to a halt with no let up.

What happens in such a situation? Your brain sends a signal and you automatically clench your muscles to control the urinary function, isn't? Likewise you have to consciously learn the subtle technique of contracting the mula bandha (root lock) located around the pelvic region, in the area between the genitals and anus, known as the perineum.

During yoga practice the challenge lies in remembering to lock the mula bandha (root lock). It is very normal to forget this aspect whilst attaining a certain posture. Many a times we tend to remember this after releasing the posture. It is necessary to control the mula bandha (root lock) throughout the practice, to stop draining the energy flow so that it stays within the body. Mula bandha (root lock), if engaged in the appropriate manner, helps to flush out toxins and also stimulate the digestive organs.

I asked my teacher as to how would I be aware if I was doing it in the right manner. "It is simple," she said. "If you get a floating sensation at the end of your session when you wake up from the final savasana (corpse pose), you are nearly there."

Engaging the mula bandha (root lock) can be quite intimidating initially but with practice we will start to feel at ease.

Uddiyana Bandha (Abdominal lock) – This body lock is located just above your navel, the belly button, and below the rib cage, where the solar plexus meridian is located. From mula bandha (root lock), the energy flows upwards to the uddiyana bandha (abdominal lock). This flow stimulates the abdominal muscles and also controls the metabolic rate of the body by helping the digestive system. The energy is then transmitted to the stomach, liver and spleen which help in toning the abdomen.

Now that we understand where this bandha (interior body lock) is located and the flow of energy, you might be wondering as to how do we engage this body lock and use it to our advantage in yoga practice.

There is a technique that I have been taught known as 'forward folds'.

- Firstly, stand erect and take a deep breath through the nose.
- Fill your belly with oxygen and then take a deep breath to fill up your lungs, in order to fully oxygenate your body.
- Whilst doing so raise your arms upwards and get ready for a forward fold. With a deep exhale, bend the waist and then come all the way down extending the bend from the hips.

- As you bend forward make sure that your neck is hanging loose and arms are dangling. This is to ensure that there is no tightness in those parts.
- Simultaneously pull in your abdominal muscles, tighten and hold the breath.

You should actually be able to see and feel the rib cage as a deep concave or hollow is formed when you contract your abdominal muscles.

- And that is not all. You are required to hold this position for as long as you can. If you find it uncomfortable, you may raise yourself a little bit, still in the forward bend, and rest both hands on your knees. You can slightly bend your knees.
- Then inhale deeply through your nose as you come into the standing position and exhale deeply as you relax.

Engaging this bandha throughout the session is urged and we must mindfully decide 'when' and 'how' to do it. Surely, this will come with practice and may take a while before it becomes an auto process. You have to start trying as soon as you get more familiar with yoga practice.

For most of us, engaging the uddiyana bandha (abdominal lock) may seem daunting. But, trust me, it is not that hard once you are guided into it by an instructor. I strongly recommend that it is best to learn the bandhas (interior body locks) from an experienced yoga teacher so that you do it the right way and reap the benefits completely. The washboard flat tummy is nearly certain if we mindfully engage this bandha (interior body lock). Can there be a better motivation to get started?

Activating your abdominal lock is also an integral part in pranayama (breathing techniques) practice. Surya namaskar (sun salutations) is one of the best series where one can learn to engage the uddiyana bandha (abdominal lock). There are forward folds in various asana (postures) where you can do so. All these have been illustrated in Part 2 of this book.

Jalandhara bandha (Throat lock) – Typically this bandha (interior body lock) is practised in pranayama (breathing techniques). How does one lock the throat?

- Sit comfortably, either cross-legged or in a half-lotus position or in vajrasana (thunderbolt pose) with both hands on your thighs.
- Inhale deeply through the nose and as you hold onto your breath, slowly bring your head down and press the chin below your neck, as if you are checking for a double chin. Stay here for as long as you can hold your breath.
- If required you can press both hands on the floor for an extra support. When you feel you can no longer hold your breath, slowly exhale and simultaneously raise your head and look straight.
- Relax the neck muscles completely and then repeat the process a few times.

Throat lock is also a part of the pranayama (breathing techniques) practice and both uddiyana (abdominal) and jalandhara (throat) bandhas (interior body locks) put together help in alleviating the sinuses, nasal blocks, softens the throat and prevents it from getting sore and tired. For those whose job entails exerting the vocal cords to extreme limits, such as receptionists, call centre employees or telephone operators, learning jalandhara bandha (throat lock) is very beneficial.

Personally, apart from the forward bending asana (postures) two other postures where I can comfortably engage all the above-mentioned interior body locks concurrently are the *halasana* (plow pose) and *sarvangasana* (shoulder stand pose).

These have been dealt with in Part 2 of this book.

Lock your bandhas and let that energy flow…

Note: Jalandhara bandha, commonly known as chin lock has been coined as throat lock as it bears an impact on the throat by locking the chin.

8

Yin and Yang

The literal meaning of yin and yang is 'shadow' and 'light', respectively. We could say that yin and yang are two sides of the same coin. They come as a bundle and are not mutually exclusive of each other. Yin is the passive stillness in a posture whereas yang is the more active, agile and energetic movement. However, the power of the two cannot be undermined. Just because yin is passive, it does not mean that it is less powerful. On the contrary, for those who desire to deepen their yoga practice, yin can be very good as it involves meditative and restorative postures.

I was introduced to this concept in the Western world. Initially I was under the mistaken impression that this variation was based on the Chinese concept of yin and yang. But as I started attending the yin classes, I understood that yin yoga involved yoga postures which had to be achieved and held for two to three minutes. Unaided holding of yin postures is not recommended by most yoga instructors and students are encouraged to use props so that they can comfortably hold the posture.

Yin yoga, founded by Paulie Zink, has blossomed uniquely with its own restorative postures which are easier to settle into. It focusses on stretching the fascia or connective tissues – tendons, ligaments and cartilage by intense stretches and then becoming still. At the same time we must focus on our breath. The postures not only help to calm the mind, but also open up the joints and make the body more supple and free by releasing the tension in the deeper connective tissues of our body. Practice of yin yoga asana (postures) along with ujjayi breathing helps the mind to be alert, concentrate and stay in the present moment. For those who find it difficult to sit in a single pose and meditate, yin yoga can be very helpful, where after meditation will become easier. Typically the sessions are conducted with soft music and candles/flowers/incense to enhance the ambience.

My instructor, Victoria, informed us that those who were unable to do active yoga practice due to health reasons (surgery or back pain and the like) could adhere to a continued and prolonged yin practice. Further, those in the 50-plus age bracket, who wanted to deepen yoga practice, could get on with yin practice alone. Yin yoga also helps in blood circulation and strengthens the tendons and ligaments which start to become dry and groan with advancement in age. Considering that these tips were coming from an instructor who had been in a terrible road accident and was successfully running a yoga studio, it was insightful and worth listening to.

Personally I find yin yoga very satisfying and rejuvenating especially after long, tedious travels. A good time to practise yin yoga is in the afternoon as the restorative postures help to wear off the mid-afternoon sluggishness.

Stillness is what I love the most in my yin practice. At a subconscious level it allows us to penetrate deep within through proper breathing and mindfulness. Yin practice also helps in improving meditation and self-awareness. This could also be a first step for those who wish to deepen their yoga practice. Yin sessions make one feel energised, positive and good about themselves and everything around them.

It must however be remembered that once we have reached

our level of endurance whilst stretching, we should simply relax, let go, stay with the breath and enjoy the stillness.

There are a few specific restorative asana (postures) that are especially designed for a yin class. These are:

- Savasana (Corpse pose)
- Supta Baddha Konasana (Supine bound angle pose)
- Sphinx and Seal pose (a modification of Bhujangasana – Cobra pose)
- Supta Virasana (Reclining Hero pose)
- Pigeon and Sleeping Swan pose
- Shoelace pose (a modification of Gomukhasana – Cow Face pose)
- Dragon pose
- Tadpole and Frog pose
- Malasana (Garland pose)
- Viparita Karani (Legs up the wall pose)

These asana (postures) have been explained and illustrated in Part 2 of this book.

We hope to become masters of our mind someday and an enriched yin practice will help us to achieve inner peace. Liberal doses of yin yoga as part of the regimen will do wonders for all age groups and for those around us as well.

"There is no fetter like illusion, no force greater than yoga, no friend greater than knowledge and no enemy greater than ego."

– Gheranda Samhita 1:4

(Courtesy: Flow Hot Yoga)

9

The Divinity of Light and Meditation

As a little girl, I used to be fascinated and curious when I saw my mother light the traditional brass lamp before she began her daily chores. I thought she was following this ritual to please God.

"Does this make God happy?" I asked her one day, to which she replied, "Yes, God will be happy. This ritual will also bring peace and prosperity and guard our home from misfortunes. Light is God and God is light," she added.

Her reply did confuse me at that time. But now when I think about it, I feel there was much truth in those simple words said to a curious little girl.

Light is indeed divine and it is widely believed that the energy in light is a force that generates and spreads goodness and a sense of well-being. Candle, incense, lamp, whatever it may be, light is an element that brings positivity and flow of energy. In its pristine form, light signifies knowledge and wisdom; on the other hand, darkness is associated with ignorance. Most religions believe in the power of light, one way or another.

Light also improves our moods. People who live in cold countries often complain about the gloomy and dreary weather. Come summer, everybody is happy to step out and soak up the sun. Don't we all ensure that our homes get plenty of sunshine? Such is the power of light! A beautiful moment, a celebration, a romantic night, a touch of warmth, a touch of class, sheer ecstasy, a sweet memory, a contemplative state; a ray of light can touch that chord to trigger off these positive emotions. This is the magic of light!

Yoga, wisdom, meditation and light are all interconnected. Light is an invitation for that cosmic energy of the universe to dwell in our surroundings. The surya namaskar (sun salutation) which activates the prana, the life force energy within us, is an adoration of Surya, the Sun God.

Further, during a yin yoga practice or meditation, candle is lit to soften the mood, to help us concentrate better and feel the positive vibrations. This has a calming effect and we feel good.

Fragranced candles make the experience of meditation pleasant and the lingering scent serves as a focal point for our mind to dwell upon and not wander. Likewise when we practise yoga in a park at the brim of dawn in anticipation of the first ray of sunlight, it is blissful to listen to the birds, amidst nature's beauty and bounty. We are so much engrossed in our daily grind that occasionally we need these reminders to be able to appreciate the natural beauty that surrounds us and makes our yoga journey so much more enjoyable.

I recall having read an interesting fact in a book by John Ittner that at Sivananda ashrams worldwide, the food served is sattvic (mild and pure). They include only those vegetables that are grown in natural sunshine and mushrooms in particular are not served, as they are grown in dark conditions (sunshine is sattvic and darkness is tamasic).

The traits or 'gunas' of nature is well explained in Chapter 14 of the *Bhagavad Gita*. This chapter reveals the wisdom of the three characteristics of nature imparted to the great warrior Arjun by Lord Krishna.

These are:

- sattva (light)
- rajas (fire)
- tamas (darkness)

A sattvic mind is calm, serene and inquisitive; a rajasic mind is fiery and craves for power; and a tamasic mind is ignorant, lazy and dull.

Renowned yogis feel the sattva, the light within themselves. The story of Buddha and the sages who have attained enlightenment have seen this eternal light that has taken them closer to God and become one with the Almighty.

I would like to conclude this chapter with my thoughts on meditation.

What is meditation and why do we meditate?

- Meditation is an observation of our mind.
- Meditation is an observation of our thoughts.
- Meditation is silence.
- Meditation is emptiness of our mind at a subconscious level.
- Meditation is seeking of the divine power within us.
- Meditation is wisdom of the mind.
- Meditation is purity of thought and action.
- Meditation is eternal bliss.
- Meditation is that moment when everything inside us comes to a standstill.
- Meditation makes us more loving, caring and compassionate.

- Meditation helps us achieve our goals in a rational manner.
- Meditation kills the naughty ego in us.
- Meditation awakens the child in us and keeps it alive.
- Meditation makes us more willing to adapt and embrace change with courage, curiosity, wisdom and devotion.
- Meditation helps to decondition our mind.

Friends, remember that light is all pervasive and spins the energy wheel in our yoga practice and meditation.

"Yoga does not remove us from the reality or responsibilities of everyday life but rather places our feet firmly and resolutely in the practical ground of experience. We don't transcend our lives; we return to the life we left behind in the hopes of something better."

– Donna Farhi

10

A Day at the Sivananda Ashram

I cannot stress enough the importance of spiritual awareness alongside yoga asana (postures) practice and meditation. Yoga practice is in itself a spiritual awakening. If you could take it further and are able to experience a simplistic way of life at an ashram, this will give an opportunity for introspection and help in understanding the essence of life. Hence we must strive to live our life to the fullest and chase our dreams like there is no tomorrow. Continuous improvement in yoga and spirituality will help us enjoy and cherish what we are blessed with.

Therefore I have included this chapter on Sivananda ashram based on my visit to the place which not only was satisfying but also had a positive impact on my life.

Rishikesh is considered to be one of the four *devlok* (abode of the gods). As per the ancient legend, it is believed that when the devas (gods) and the asuras (demons) were at combat churning the ocean, each hopeful of winning the eternal nectar, four drops accidentally fell on *Bhoomadevi* (Mother Earth). One drop fell on this spot and therefore Rishikesh is considered to be a heaven on Earth, surrounded by the resplendent Himalayan range that cradles the mighty Ganges – that runs alongside the ashram.

A day at the ashram begins at 5.00 a.m. with prayer and chants followed by meditation at the Swami Sivananda Samadhi Shrine and concludes with a short talk in English. What a different way to start a morning! There may be quite a few of you who start the day with meditation but there is always a nagging thought of "what if the milkman or paperboy rings the doorbell," and this can be pretty distracting. At the ashram, it is a different ambience with pin-drop silence except for the occasional chirping of the birds or the rustle of leaves. Thereafter chants of *'Om Namah Shivaya'* echo in the air with devotees sitting quietly with eyes closed and being in the moment. The harmonium (a wind musical instrument) adds a zing to the chorus chanting. This is followed by the divine *mangala aarti* (prayer and offering) to Lord Shiva and other deities.

Soon after that I heard the sound of a bell. I realised that it was time for breakfast as I saw everyone walk towards the dining hall. Lunch and dinner are likewise served sharp at 11.30 a.m. and 7.00 p.m. after a short prayer to thank the Lord for his kindness.

Ashram food is free for not only the ashramites but for visitors, as well. To express gratitude, devotees take part in kitchen duties like cutting veggies and serving food. Swami Sivananda's abiding principle that no work is menial could be adequately seen in the mix of devotees who took part in kitchen duties.

The food served at the ashram is sattvic. Sattvic food is a healthy vegetarian meal with low salt diet and spices just enough to make the food tasty. Spicy food like pickles and chillies (rajasic) that can make us agitated and angry; and heavy food (tamasic) including meat is not something you will find here. You would be surprised to know that the ashram does not serve coffee. Only tea is made available. This is because caffeine can interfere with meditation.

The general library and audio-visual library have an amazing and vast collection of books on spirituality, Eastern and Western philosophy, yoga, scriptures and many other interesting topics, apart from the collection of books and lectures by Swami Sivananda and his disciples. It was a delight to spend a few quiet afternoons there.

The evening satsang from 7.30 p.m. to 9.30 p.m. at the Samadhi Shrine was pure bliss. After the opening prayer and recitations from the scripture, devotees are encouraged to sing bhajans and kirtans followed by a lecture on spirituality or audio-visuals of his disciples as they addressed devotees around the globe.

I never missed my walk to Gurudev *Kutir* (Gurudev's house) which is on the banks of the Ganges. This was where Swami Sivananda lived. His entire belongings including the furniture, medals and trophies have been well preserved. Even the tiles remain unchanged and the marble flooring has aged well over time. His life story has been portrayed in paintings and sculptures.

I would choose a spot on the banks of the Ganges and recall stories that I have heard from my grandmother. It felt as if every legend was a reality and not a myth and the characters would literally come alive before my eyes. I used to drift into my own world of imagination and joy. What we see on the internet does only half justice to the scenic beauty of this place.

No wonder, devotees and seekers from all over the world come to this part in search of their spiritual self. It was amazing to meet and bond with devotees from Switzerland, Japan, Italy, England and Netherlands as well as from Mumbai, Chennai, Bengaluru and many other parts of India. This indeed was 'unity in diversity'.

With each passing day I started to feel a sense of involvement, physically, mentally and emotionally, towards the ashram routine. I could feel the vibrancy in the air and the resplendent surroundings added to the divinity. Although, initially, I found it challenging to keep pace with the recitation of the verses from Hindu scriptures, in less than a week, I had started making progress and was able to participate more meaningfully.

This is a gentle reminder to us all that practice is the key to learning.

This visit was my baby step in the divine path of spirituality and I have a long way to go. Learning, understanding, adapting and evolving makes life more interesting. If a two-week stay can endow so much bliss, joy, positivity, peace and renewed energy, just imagine how life would be if we chase material comforts along with an awareness of self and spirituality?

This ashram set amidst the majestic Himalayas is undoubtedly a heaven on earth – devloka in this *kaliyug*.

Part 2 – Asana (Postures)

{Explanations with Illustrations}

11

Introduction

We are what we eat – say health experts.

We are what we think – say philosophers.

We are what we do – say holistic health gurus.

Do you notice the commonality of 'We' in the above?

"What do you want in life?"

Most of us would list happiness as our first choice.

But in order to be happy we need…and our wish list begins. It may differ from one person to another. The route may vary but the end result is that we all desire happiness.

By and large most of us would agree that in order to be happy and stay that way we need good health, a successful career to help us achieve our goals, a happy home and family, material comfort, peace and so on. Money is something everybody, including a spiritual person, needs to survive.

People who are successful in the material world are not necessarily unhappy if they are able to balance their material pursuit along with spiritual awareness. As long as money power is a means to an end and not an end by itself, a person can still be content and happy. There is nothing wrong about having materialistic needs. It is only when desire turns into avarice and brings out the monster in us that it gets disastrous. Happiness lies within us and we need to realise and understand this truth in our own way.

The eight fold path of yoga, as described in the yoga sutras (aphorisms) by sage Patanjali, is one of the tools to achieve this state of mind. The path comprises the following:

- Yama (Social discipline or the abstinences) – It entails social virtues such as *ahimsa* (non-violence), *satya* (truth), *asteya* (non-stealing), *brahmacharya* (continence) and *aparigraha* (non-covetousness) and to be able to blend with the norms of society and civilised living.
- Niyama (Individual discipline or the observances) – It entails individual qualities such as *saucha* (purity in words and deed), *santosha* (contentment), *tapas* (austerity), *svadhyaya* (study or knowledge of oneself) and *ishvar pranidhana* (love towards your deity) and becoming a better person.
- Asana (Postures) – It deals with the physical aspects of yoga.
- Pranayama (Regulated breathing) – It deals with the various breathing techniques in order to improve concentration and meditative practices.
- Pratyahara (Mind being able to control the senses) – It requires prolonged practice of meditation to be able to see things the way they are, without being judgmental or contemplative, and to reach your pure inner self.
- Dharana (Concentration) – It means being able to achieve oneness with your mind, no matter where you are or in what surrounding you may be.
- Dhyana (Meditation) – This is the level where you are able to control both mind and body and stay in a blissful state of emptiness and nothingness.
- Samadhi (Enlightenment) – This is the stage where your soul leaves your body and transmigrates and becomes one with the Supreme power.

If we are able to put to practice the first four limbs of yoga, the rest will eventually follow over time, depending on how diligent and persevering we are with our practice. As mentioned earlier, it could take a lifetime or even beyond.

This is what differentiates the common man and the seers and saints who have been able to achieve samadhi (enlightenment) in their lifetime.

Yogacharya B.K.S. Iyengar in his book, *Yoga Wisdom & Practice* (for health, happiness and a better world) makes a lovely analogy of these eight limbs of yoga to parts of a mango tree.

He says that "the eight aspects of yoga are like a gigantic mango tree which starts from the seed to the root, root to the trunk, trunk to the branches, branches sprouting into leaves, leaves aerating the entire tree supplying energy in the form of sap through the bark, and later blossom into flowers culminating with tasty fruit."

In order to keep our mind active, rational, strong, sane and healthy, we need the support of our body and vice versa. All yoga asana (postures) have overall health benefits. They tend to stimulate the various glands, adrenals, gonads and meridians in our body. This improves immunity, stamina, concentration and agility, and makes us less prone to sickness and diseases. However, this does not mean that we will not be afflicted by a viral infection or we will not have flu or sore throat or stomach upsets or such irritants. Yoga practice will help us overcome these and make us less prone to common ailments. We also learn to remain positive under adverse circumstances.

I cannot therefore stress enough the importance of knowing and understanding our mind and body. Some of you may be familiar with the yoga postures and its health benefits. This part of the book would serve as a refresher to those who are already into yoga practice and as a learning guide to those who are getting their foothold into yoga.

In this part, I have included various asana (postures) which if practised regularly can enhance self-awareness and also help to deepen your yoga practice.

Please remember that it is not really important as to the number of postures you can achieve or perfect, as long as you are able to follow a few and slowly add a few more but keep practising diligently, till your body is ready to pick up some more asana (postures) along the way. There is an initial adjustment period which needs to be recognised and understood. Therefore it is advisable to start with simple postures that also have equally good health benefits as compared to the more challenging postures.

In this part an attempt has been made to cover a wide range of asana (postures), with stepwise details and illustrations that are easy to grasp and adhere to. It starts with the surya namaskar (sun salutation) sequence followed by supine, prone, seated and standing postures.

Note: A word of caution for readers with health issues: The benefits of each asana (posture) has been dealt with from a holistic perspective. Please consult your doctor and make sure to choose the postures that suit you the most.

12

Surya Namaskar (Sun Salutation) Sequence

1. Tadasana (Mountain Pose)

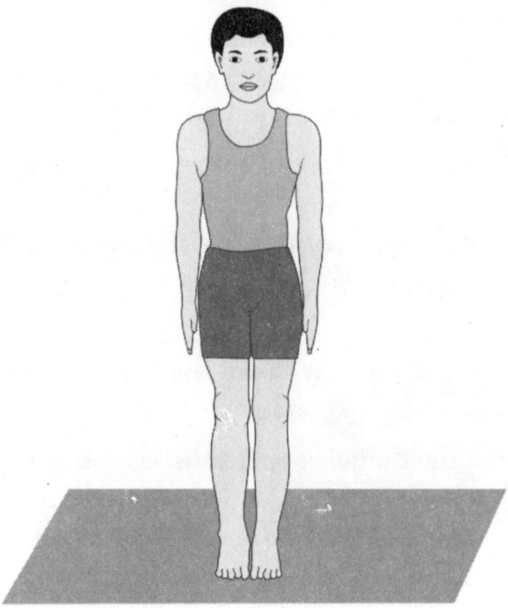

This is the rudimentary standing pose, also known as *samasthiti*, from where the sun salutation sequence begins. True to its terminology, this asana (posture) is meant to be performed in a majestic manner and the challenge lies in keeping still, firm, solid as a rock but at the same time being able to relax the entire body, maintaining a soft, rhythmic breath with total awareness of it.

Steps

a) Stand erect with feet placed together. The sole of the feet should be pressed on the floor and the toes should feel the yoga mat.

b) Keep your back and spine erect, shoulders straight and aligned to your hips, neck firm and arms on either side, close to the body with fingers, active and pointing to the floor.

c) Look ahead and hold your gaze steady. Letting the eyes wander will disturb the equilibrium of the stance.

d) Close your eyes and take a deep, slow breath to inhale and then exhale in the same manner. Focus on your breathing as your abdomen rises and falls and maintain this pose.

   Stay still and rooted to the ground and feel your body get lighter as if Mother Earth is bearing the entire body weight. In your mind you may thank Jagat Janani (Mother Earth) for supporting your stance.

   It is important to relax your muscles and not tighten any part of the body. Firmness, not tautness, is vital to this posture. Stand tall like the majestic Himalayas and breathe in the pure air. As you exhale, bring out all the toxins and impurities within you. Take a few breaths and feel rejuvenated.

   Hold this position for at least a minute to feel at ease. Join both hands in anjali (prayer position) and get ready to start the sun salutation series.

Benefits

This contemplative posture calms the mind and helps concentration as well as body balance. This asana (posture) strengthens the muscles and stimulates the meridians in our body. All the minute details have to be taken care whilst in the stance, in order to reap the benefits. Stillness, steadiness and focus are crucial and this combination is not easy in the initial stages. You need to tame your mind and body to make this asana (posture) work for you. It also prepares you to begin the sun salutation sequence.

2. Urdhva Hastasana (Raised Hands Pose)

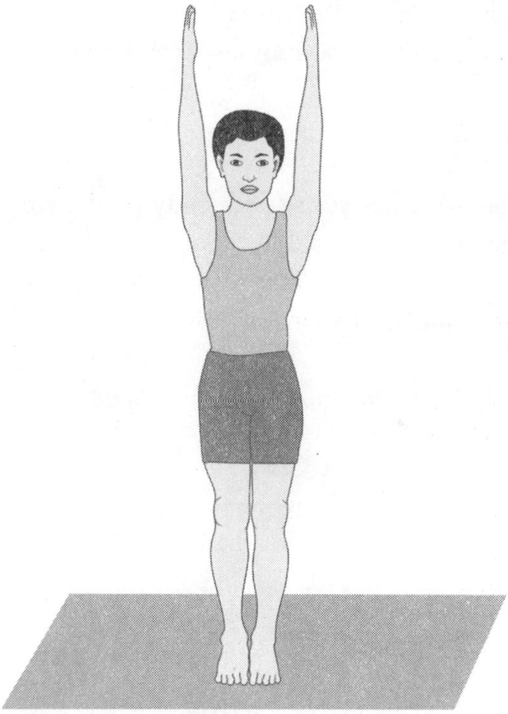

Steps

a) From tadasana (mountain pose), take a deep inhalation. Please remember that the oceanic powerful breath known as ujjayi breath will hold you in good stead if you practise it with each and every movement.

b) As you inhale, engage the mula bandha (root lock) and raise both arms upwards above your head. You may join palms in anjali (prayer position). Feel the stretch at your waist, chest and shoulders.

c) Gently shift your gaze up at your palms. This would arch your back slightly, but that is meant to be so. Care should be taken to not tighten the buttocks. The gluteus should be very relaxed. Breathe for a few seconds. In this position your shoulders will eventually touch your ears, without any strain to the neck muscles. Please do not fret if it does not.

Benefits

This posture stretches your entire body particularly the upper body, opens up your shoulder joints, and promotes stability and body balance. It also creates mobility in your rib cage and enables the spine for the next intense forward bend.

3. Uttanasana (Forward Bend Pose)

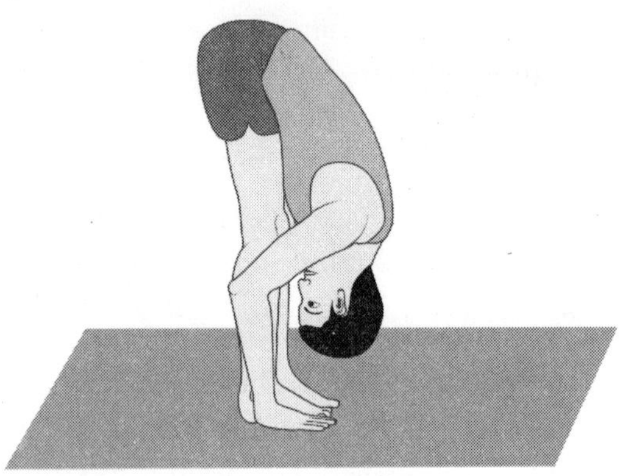

Steps

a) Take a deep inhalation and as you exhale, extend your

body forward from the hips. Release your palms from the prayer position and bring arms together with your upper torso to follow this movement. Then bend all the way down. Remember to engage your uddiyana bandha (abdominal lock) and mula bandha (root lock), as you fold forward.

b) Bring your head downwards with the crown almost touching the floor.

c) Try and shift your body weight to the balls of your feet as this will help you bend a bit more. Your gaze will automatically rest at a point between your legs. That is your focus or *drishti*.

d) You could try and hold both ankles and bring your head closer in-between the legs, as much as you can and then rest both palms as shown in the illustration. However, do not taut your neck muscles and remember to keep your head and neck freely hanging and loose.

   In the final stage of this asana (posture), you will be able to lock your jalandhara bandha (throat lock) as well. Enjoy and take a few breaths here. Adjust your body alignment to stay comfortable and feel the renewed energy in your solar plexus in this inverted pose.

Benefits

This is an intense stretch for the spine and the back that makes them very supple and flexible.

It also helps to tone the thigh and calf muscles. As in all other inversion postures, it helps in supply of oxygen to the brain and nerve cells and improves vision and hearing. This is an extremely therapeutic posture if you are able to hold it for a few minutes.

4. Lunge

(a)

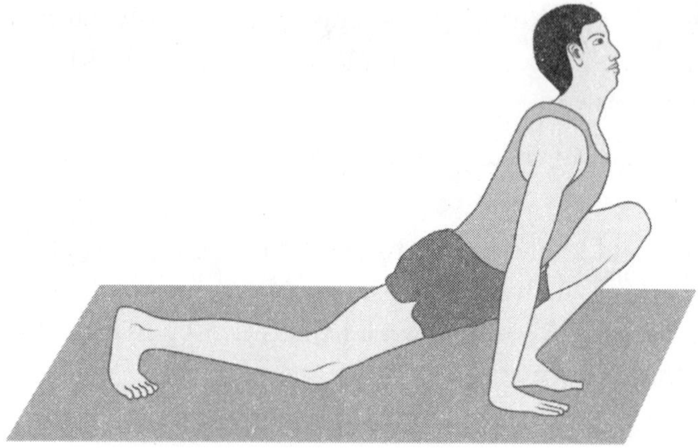

(b)

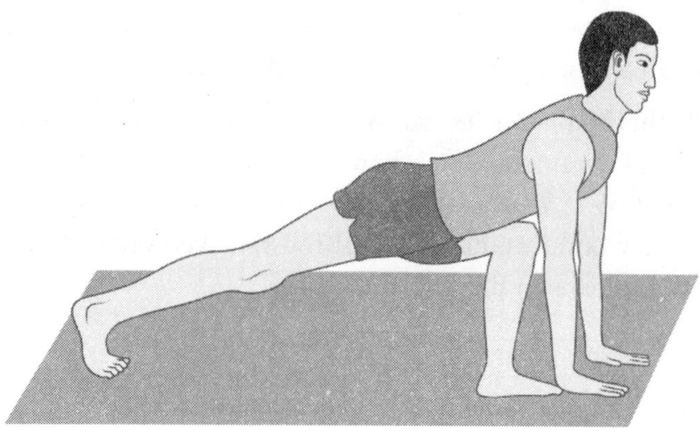

This is an intermediary position that helps you to get into the next asana (posture) which is the four-limbed high plank pose. The illustration in (a) is the traditional recommended posture for beginners. Some prefer a minor variation to this lunge, by trying to not rest the right knee on the floor, instead keeping it straight, as illustrated in (b). You may follow either of the two.

Steps

a) Inhale and extend your right leg backwards. Bend the right knee to touch the floor and curl your toes.
b) Left knee is to be placed close to the chest, with the thigh supporting your chest.
c) Press both hands to the floor on either side of the left foot and relax your facial and neck muscles. Exhale.

Benefits

This posture is a good stretch for the legs especially the quadriceps, hamstrings and calves as well as the pelvic muscles. It is also a preparatory posture and helps you to relax a bit after the intense forward fold to move on to the next asana (posture), the four-limbed high plank pose, which is a very powerful posture.

Yoga experts who are more experienced release their hold on the ankles and, with both hands pressed on the floor, directly jump into four-limbed high plank pose straight from uttanasana (forward bend pose). But this needs precision, balance, core strength and muscle power. The energy that is generated in uttanasana helps them to take this swift jump.

I would recommend that you follow the lunge variations because surya namaskar (sun salutation) is meant to be done with a steady amount of dynamism. Occasionally you can try jumping straight into high plank pose just to test your energy levels.

5. Four-limbed High Plank Pose

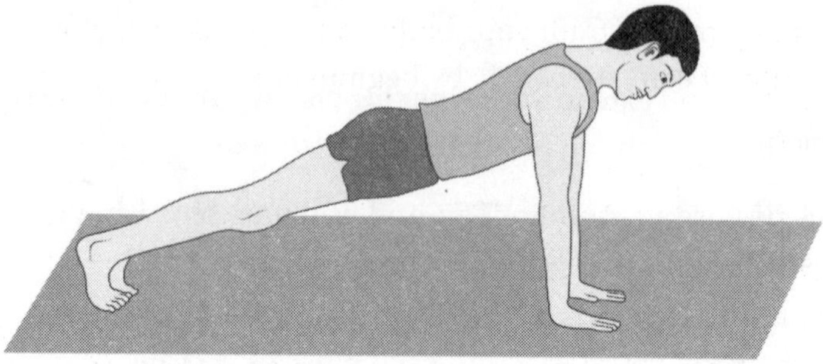

This is one of the stimulating postures in the series as it challenges as well as strengthens your core muscles. I can't emphasise enough how important this posture is to develop and improve your core strength. The core muscles are the fulcrum which holds the entire trunk of our body. The six packs is something which most youngsters rave about these days. Even women love to have their core under control.

Steps

a) With a deep inhalation extend your left leg backwards from lunge position and keep both legs straight and steady and curl your toes. Squeeze the abdomen muscles but relax your gluteus.

b) Straighten your arms, rotate and open up both shoulders. Firmly press the palms on the floor. Your shoulders, elbows and wrists should be in a straight line.

c) Raise your body above the floor using your arm and core strength and look down. In this position your head, back and legs should be aligned. Your body weight rests on your arms, balls of the feet and toes.

   If you decide to jump directly from uttanasana (forward bend pose), take a deep inhalation and pressing both palms on the floor on either side of the feet, extend legs backwards in a quick movement. Please be aware that this jump might strain your body and so it has to be done with utmost care, especially by beginners.

Benefits

This posture strengthens core and arm muscles and tones your legs. This is also a perfect posture to improve your agility.

6. Chaturanga Dandasana (Four-limbed Staff Pose)

(a)

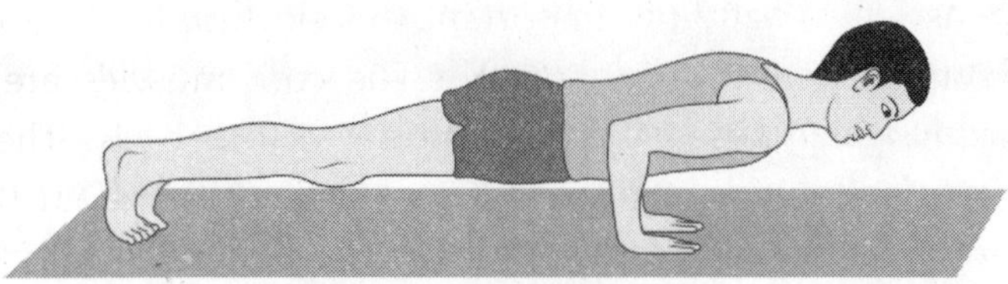

(b) Intermediary asana

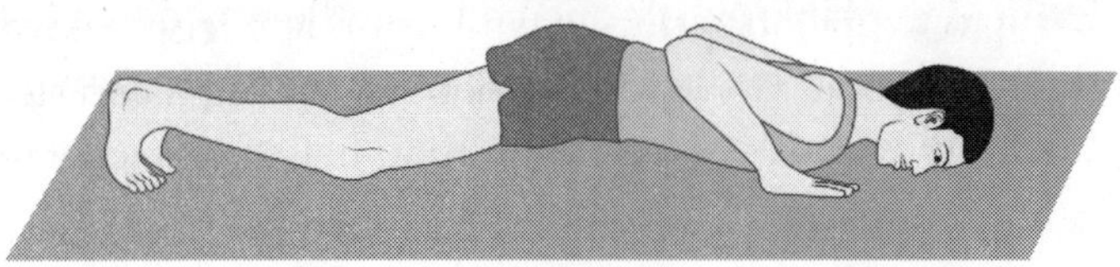

This asana (posture) can be done in two ways, as illustrated above.

Steps for (a)

a) From high plank, exhale and come down to chaturanga dandasana (four-limbed staff pose) or low plank. This is an intense posture. You are still above the floor; the chest and rest of the body are to be held a few inches away from the floor.

b) You are required to bend your elbows symmetrical to your body and balance on the strength of the arm muscles as you push your body downwards. The body is like a straight stick suspended a few inches above the floor.

c) Please make sure you open up the shoulders and allow your elbows and palms to be positioned as depicted in the figure.

Suggestion

You may find this chaturanga dandasana (four-limbed staff pose) extremely challenging unless you have been practising press-ups or push-ups. The risk is that the knees might collapse or you may involuntarily let the belly sag. Both are not desirable as it might hurt your shoulders or back. Hence unless you are ready for it, I would urge you to use the intermediary posture as shown in illustration (b).

Steps for (b)

a) From high plank, exhale and come all the way down to the floor with your buttocks raised, knees lightly touching the floor and toes curled.

b) Stomach and abdomen should be above the floor. Control your abdominal muscles and do not tighten the buttocks.

   This is an easier alternative highly recommended for beginners.

Benefits

This posture builds and strengthens your core muscles, legs and arms and the intermediary posture is also beneficial in balancing your body and preparing for the next asana (posture) which is an intense backbend.

7. Urdhva Mukha Svanasana (Upward Facing Dog Pose)

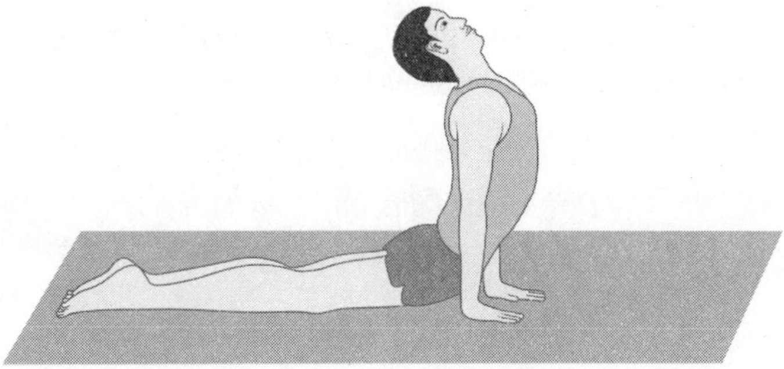

This is an intense backbend.

Steps

a) With a deep inhalation raise your upper body and arch it backwards, as much as you can and look up.

b) Open up your shoulder joints and push your chest forward as you inhale and bend backwards, so that you do not strain your wrists or arms and are able to balance your body evenly. Do not bend the elbows.

c) In this position, the abdomen must not touch the floor. The upper body curves backwards shifting the body weight to the lower half and arms. You will feel your thighs, groin and knees touch the floor. Your legs should be rooted to the ground, steady and straight with toes toggled together.

   Breathe evenly. Take few breaths here and engage your mula bandha (root lock).

Benefits

This is a contra pose to the next asana (posture) which is the downward facing dog pose and is an excellent backbend.

It strengthens the spine and improves elasticity. This asana (posture) also stretches the entire upper body and opens up the chest. It releases tension in the shoulder joints and neck and tones the leg muscles, as well.

8. Adho Mukha Svanasana (Downward Facing Dog Pose)

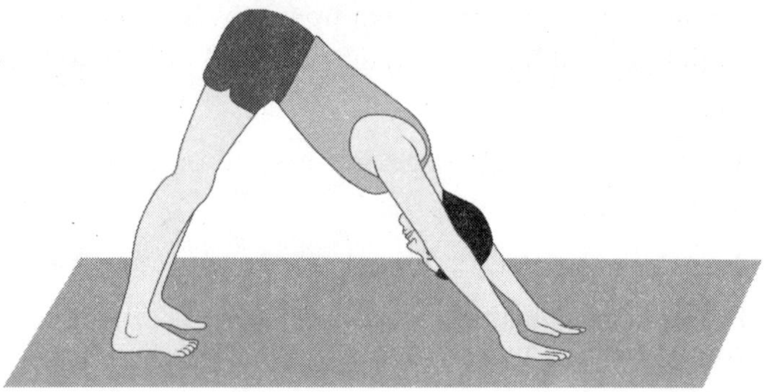

This is a beautiful inversion posture and contra to the upward facing dog pose. Thus far you have taken a couple of breaths in the earlier posture. Your body has sufficiently stretched and warmed up and fully geared to come to this down dog posture with more spirit and enthusiasm. Please do remember to take it easy if this is your first down dog pose for the day.

Steps

a) From upward facing dog pose take a deep inhalation and inch backwards in a frog like position, resting buttocks on the heels. As you exhale lift your body up to attain an inverted V. Try to simultaneously activate your uddiyana bandha (abdominal lock).

b) The stretch has to be from the hips. Make sure your tail

bone points upwards and keep adjusting your legs so that you can comfortably balance your upper body in the manner described.

c) Your hands should be firmly pressed on the floor and face should be in-between your arms, with the crown almost touching the floor. Keep the neck and head loose and hanging without any strain. Adjust and rotate your shoulders so as to open them up nicely. Elbows should be straight so that the body weight is evenly distributed on all four limbs.

d) The spine should be erect and this is possible if you keep lifting your tail bone upwards.

e) Transfix your drishti (gaze) on your abdomen or any point above or below your navel, wherever you feel comfortable. This will help you focus and sink into the asana (posture).

f) Lock your mula bandha (root lock) and tuck your chin inwards to rest, just below the hollow of your neck, and lock the jalandhara bandha (throat lock) as well.

   As in all inversion postures you will feel the facial muscles getting massaged and your cheeks becoming fuller. Take a couple of breaths in this position.

Suggestion

A little adjustment may be required for those with tight hamstrings. You could shift your weight from one foot to another, bend knees slightly and balance on the balls of your feet.

Benefits

This posture massages the internal digestive organs and ensures fresh supply of oxygen to the brain. Apart from strengthening the four limbs it also makes your spine strong and flexible. This posture increases the stamina of the body by removing energy blockages. This is an excellent posture where you can lock all the three bandhas (interior body locks) and energise.

9.Lunge

(a)

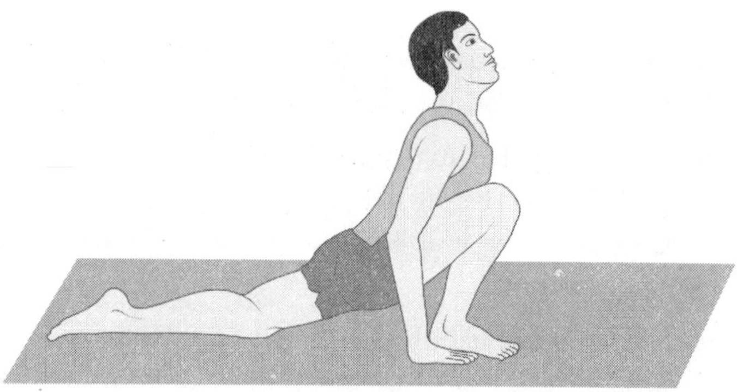

(b)

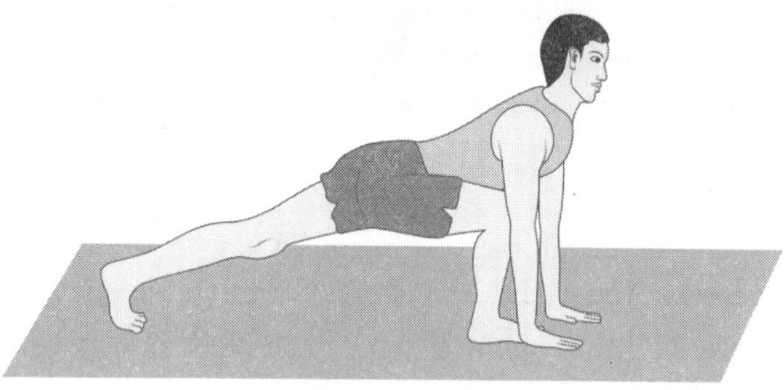

This is the same as described earlier, except that now you bring the right leg forward, in a lunge position, as shown above.

10. Uttanasana (Forward Bend Pose)

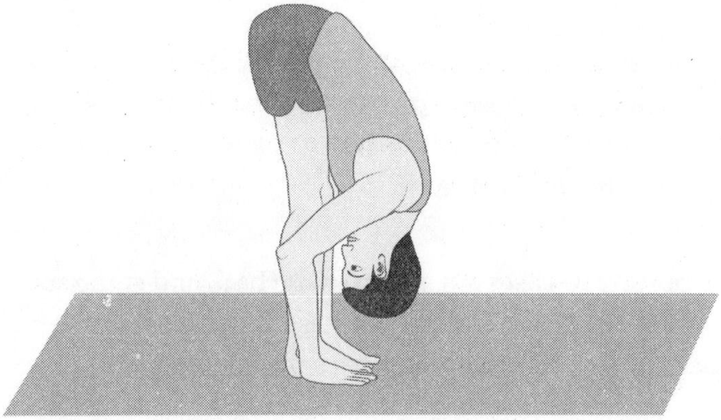

This has been explained earlier and hence the explanation has not been repeated here.

11. Intense Backbend Pose

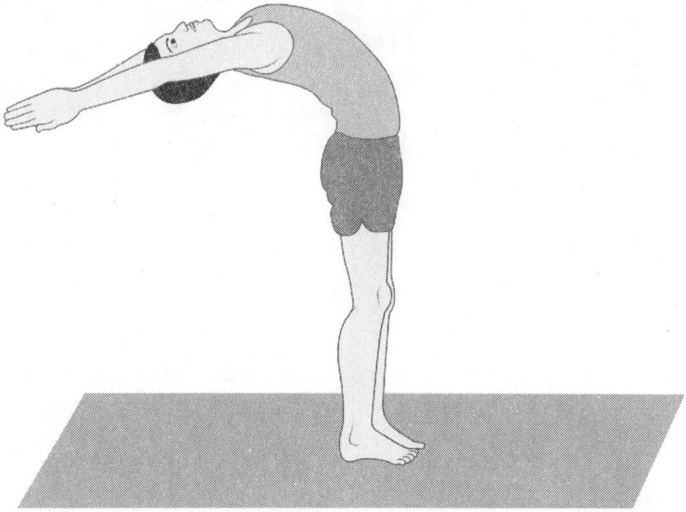

This is a contra pose to uttanasana (forward bend pose) and helps to relax the back before coming back to the original stance, tadasana (mountain pose).

Steps

a) Take a deep inhalation and come all the way up from the forward bend pose to an extended backbend pose.
b) Keep hands in prayer position or parallel to each other and remember to breathe.

Benefits

This posture releases any strain in the back and spine and also creates space in the rib cage. It has all the merits of a frontal upper body stretch as it stimulates the energy points.

12. Tadasana (Mountain Pose)

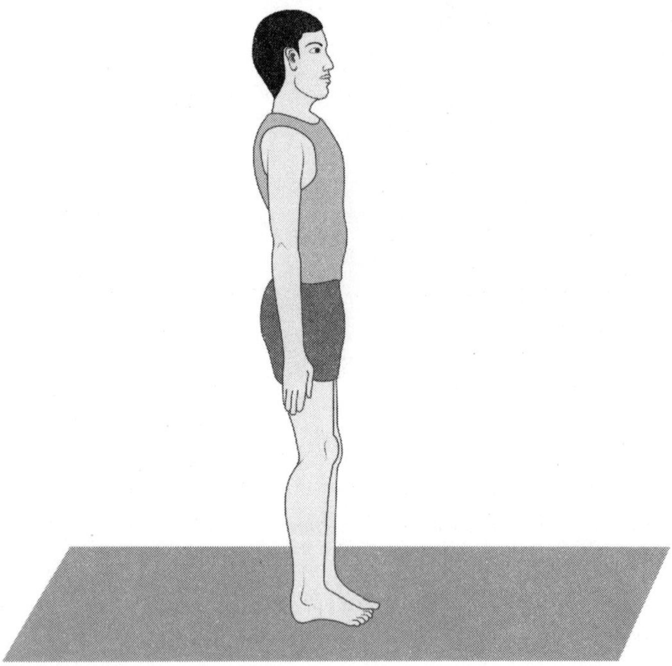

Come back to the start position, tadasana (mountain pose) on an exhale.

Conclusion

This series can be repeated as many times as you wish. Start with three to six times and gradually increase to ten or twelve rounds. Practice with grace and fervour as this is an invocation of the Sun God.

Tips

As a general rule, while practising any posture it is encouraged to extend that limb of your body which you move in order to feel the maximum stretch. For example, in urdhva hastasana (raised hands pose) try to extend from your shoulders and reach out upwards and do not loosely raise your arms. Only then will you feel the full stretch.

There is nothing like 'rush' or 'perfect' in yoga. Your practice is exclusive. Allow the body to show you how to advance in each and every posture. It is always good to understand the ground rules from the initial stages of practice. Remember that everybody started off as a beginner someday.

Note

After uttanasana (forward bend pose) some instructors urge to take the downward facing dog posture before coming to high plank pose. These sort of minor variations are introduced to help people with different body conditions.

13

Supine Postures
(Lying on the back)

The yoga asana (postures) can be broadly classified under four heads:

- Supine postures – lying on the back
- Prone Postures – lying on the belly
- Seated postures
- Standing postures

In this chapter, I have explained the various asana (postures) that would be good to begin with and also aid in a guided practice. It should be remembered that for every posture there is a contra pose that is necessary to be followed, so as to maintain the equilibrium and avoid straining the body in one direction alone. This has also been explained at appropriate places.

The first set of asana (postures) that is required to be done lying on the back comprises the following:

1) Savasana (Corpse pose)
2) Supta Baddha Konasana (Supine Bound Ankle pose)
3) Ananda Balasana (Happy Baby pose)
4) Viparita Karani (Legs up the Wall pose)
5) Jathara Parivartanasana (Belly Twist pose)
6) Pavanamuktasana (Wind Relieving pose)
7) Anantasana (Lying Sideways and Leg Lift pose)

8) Naukasana (Boat pose)
9) Setu Bandhasana (Bridge pose)
10) Halasana (Plow pose)
11) Matsyasana (Fish pose)
12) Urdhva Dhanurasana (Wheel pose)
13) Supta Virasana (Reclining Hero pose)
14) Sarvangasana (Shoulder Stand pose)

1. Savasana (Corpse Pose)

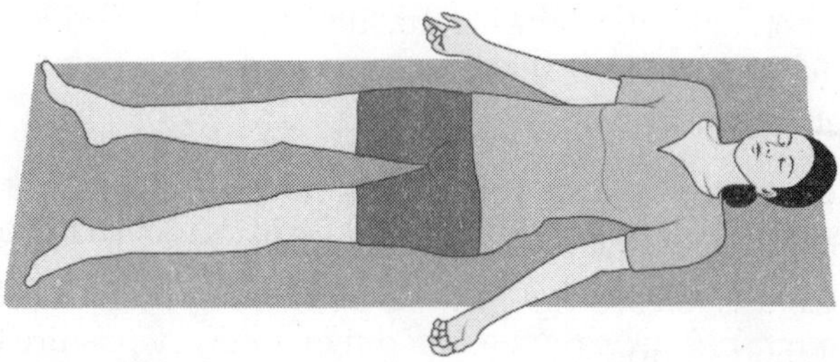

This is the basic relaxation posture. Savasana (corpse pose) relaxes your body and calms the mind. Hence typically this pose is done at the start and also at the end of a class, to rest and cool down the body. At the same time, if you feel tired during a session, it is best to come to this pose for a few seconds and then get back into action.

Steps

a) Lie down still, with arms by your side and palms facing upwards to draw the cosmic energy. Bring both legs close together and let them slide apart with toes tilting naturally on either side. This may feel awkward and passive but it is the perfect pose to start the relaxation process by focussing your attention and breath on each and every part of the body and achieving a sense of calm.

b) The spine should be kept straight and not curved. You may use a pillow as a prop and place it vertically to support your spine and lower back. Activate your bandhas (interior body locks).

Breathe evenly with eyes closed, lips sealed and tongue resting under the edge of your upper jaw or wherever you feel comfortable. Resting the tongue is only to control your saliva and avoid jerks whilst swallowing it. Listen to your heart beats.

The moment you are expected to be still is the time you get that sudden urge to wiggle your toes or scratch the forehead or ears. This is very common. Training the mind helps to ignore all these irritants and not break the deep spell in this posture.

The experience that you should have here is as if Mother Earth is carrying your weight and the body is floating on it. Gently release the posture by turning over to one side and then sit up.

Benefits

The posture relaxes your body, conserves energy and centres your mind. It helps in concentration and meditation.

2. Supta Baddha Konasana (Supine Bound Ankle Pose)

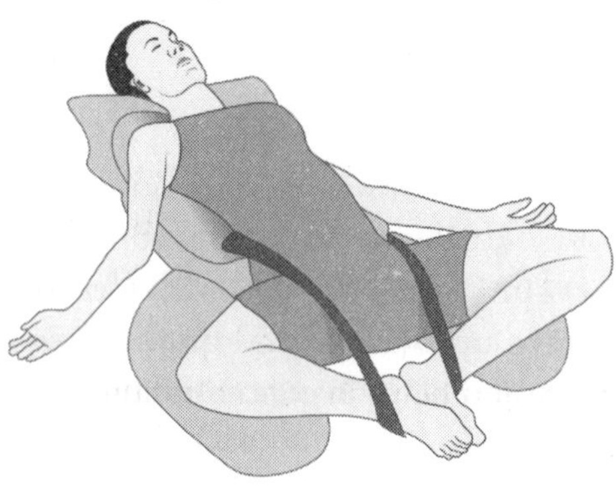

This is also a relaxation and restorative posture similar to the corpse pose.

Steps

a) Lie down and bend the knees drawing both legs close such that the soles of your feet are together.

b) Knees should be as close as possible to the floor. It might help to place two cushions to support both knees, initially, as shown in the illustration.

c) Instead of resting your arms alongside with palms facing upwards, you could rest your left hand on your chest to feel the heart beat and your right hand can gently rest on the navel.

The other steps are similar to savasana (corpse pose) and hence not repeated here.

Release the posture by stretching your legs first. Take a deep breath and stretch both arms over your head. Flex your feet, inwards and outwards, exhale and relax. Turn over to one side and sit up.

Benefits

This asana (posture) stretches your pelvic muscles and inner thighs and opens up the hips and groins. This is also a very calming posture and helps in concentration.

3. Ananda Balasana (Happy Baby Pose)

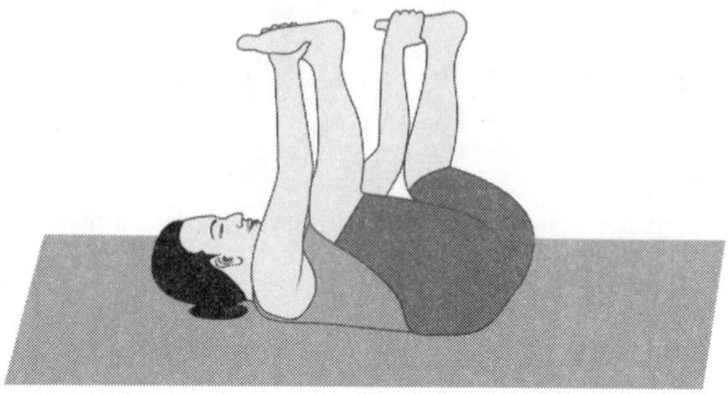

As the name suggests, this is a very enjoyable and amusing asana (posture) and can literally make you laugh as you get into it. Imagine that special childhood photo of you, lying on the back and sucking the big toe or simply holding your toes and legs bouncing like a rubber ball, so full of giggles, and at that precise moment the shutter bug clicks. Moment captured, picture framed and proud parents put it up for display. Yes! One happy baby we all were.

Steps

a) In the lying down position take a deep breath and bend your knees pushing them sideways wide apart.

b) Hold the sole of both feet from inwards, with your hands.

c) Gently push your feet downwards as if to bring the thigh parallel to the floor. Breathe out.

d) Sway from side to side, relax and enjoy like a happy baby.

e) Release the posture by coming back to savasana (corpse pose).

Benefits

This is a joyful and restorative pose that helps in improving the elasticity of legs, stretches the inner thighs, hamstrings and pelvic muscles and opens up the groins and hips. It also stimulates your digestive system.

4. Viparita Karani (Legs up the Wall Pose)

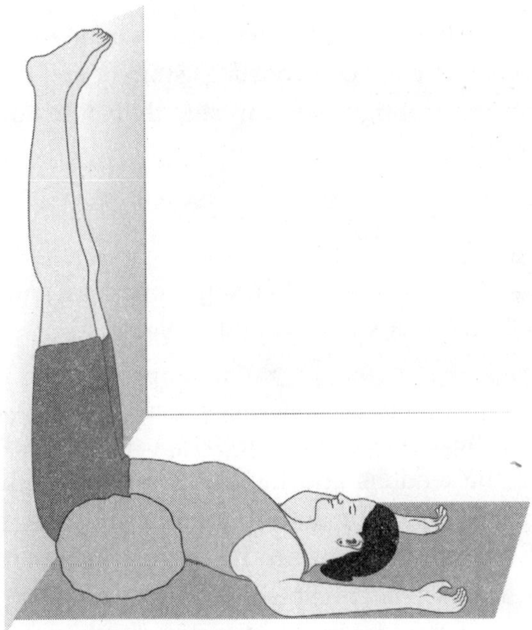

This is an easy and comfortable inversion pose and is beneficial for those with tight hamstrings.

Steps

a) Lie down sideways such that your buttocks touch the wall. As shown in the illustration you can use a bolster or simply fold two blankets to support your lower back. Alternatively, you can keep both hands tucked in just below the waist to prop up your sit bones, with palms touching the floor.

b) Take a deep inhalation and slowly raise one leg up the wall perpendicular to the body. Your other leg will be resting on the floor as in x axis mode. Exhale.

c) Take another deep inhalation and slowly raise the other leg up the wall. Both legs will be parallel to one another.

   Flex your feet and keep it active. Exhale.

   Adjust the blankets or bolster so that you feel comfortable. It is preferable to keep your legs straight and stretched. If hamstrings feel tight you can slightly bend your knees to avoid pain.

d) Close your eyes, visualise a waterfall, breathe evenly and relax in this posture.

   Release the posture by bending your legs and bringing them to the floor sideways and sit up.

Benefits

This is a gentle and easy-to-do asana (posture) which helps in exercising the tendons and ligaments and strengthens your thighs, hamstrings, calf and abdominal muscles, back and spine. This restorative posture has a very calming effect on the mind. This will later help you in halasana (plow pose) and sarvangasana (shoulder stand pose) and all other unsupported leg raise, by strengthening your backbone and core muscles.

5. Jathara Parivartanasana (Belly Twist Pose)

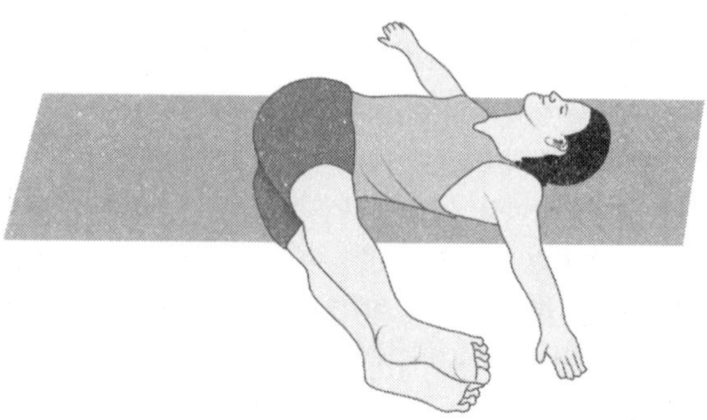

This is a challenging asana (posture) and it will take time to get this right unless you have very strong abdominal muscles. For those who have had babies, this is the best asana (posture) to get back in shape. You can use a prop belt to hold your feet in this position. However this posture may not be ideal if you have problems with your back.

Steps:

a) Lie down with legs close together and arms stretched on both sides. Take a deep inhalation. As you exhale lift both legs straight without bending at the knees, until they are perpendicular to your body. Try to use your abdominal strength and not shoulder support. If your hamstrings are tight, then slightly bend your knees. If you feel pressure in the back region, prop up a pillow or cushion to slightly lift your lower back as this will also help in the leg raise.

b) Inhale and with a deep exhalation, slowly and steadily lower both legs to the left side of the body. The legs should be held close together. Only the abdomen and waist ought to twist as you settle down in this position. Please do not turn your entire body in an attempt to get the leg position right. You may keep a chair to rest your feet initially, in case you are unable to bring your legs down on the floor, but eventually try to do away with the chair.

   Further, when you lower your legs the tendency will be to separate them as you will feel the pressure in your abdominal muscles and lower back, but try not to. Therefore be very careful whilst lowering your legs. Any sort of pain is an indicator that you are not doing it right or you need to adjust your props. Please treat the pain as a warning signal.

c) Your upper body has to be rooted to the ground. Initially the shoulders will also rise above the floor level. But try to keep them pinned down.

d) Take another deep inhalation and lift both legs together and bring them at right angle position again and as you exhale lower both legs to the right side of the body.

   Repeat this three times on both sides and then bring both the legs perpendicular to the body and lower them to start position on an exhale. Relax in savasana (corpse pose).

   If this is too hard, instead of raising the legs to repeat on the opposite side, you can also just drag both legs on the floor, all the way to the opposite side. After having done this, you have no choice but to now lift both legs up at right angle and slowly bring them back to the left side once again. This helps to marginally reduce the intensity for beginners. Repeat on the other side in the same manner.

Benefits

This is an excellent twist at the waist, hips and abdomen. This asana (posture) also strengthens your abdominal muscles and spine and tones your legs. It is also known to be a waist trimmer as it helps to shave off the flab, love handles and folds that may have developed after childbirth.

6. *Pavanamuktasana (Wind Relieving Pose)*

(a)

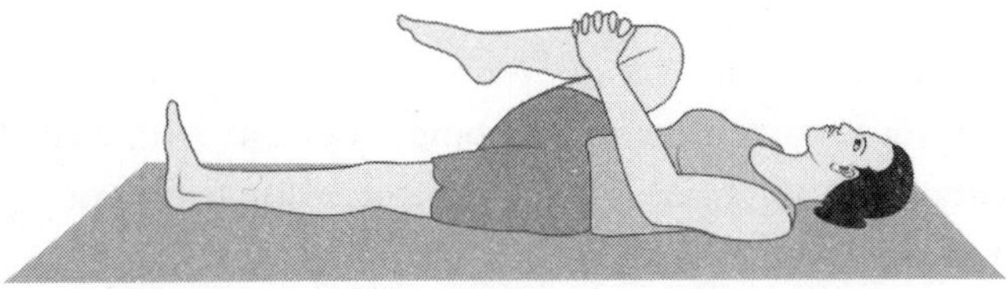

(b)

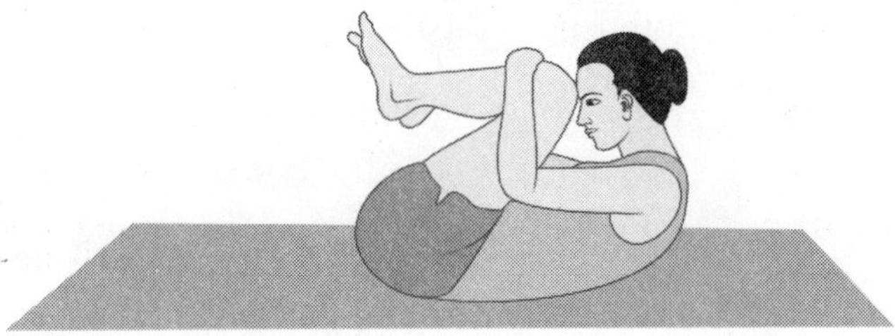

This is a relatively easy and comfortable pose. As the name suggests this is an excellent asana (posture) for those with gastric issues, as it massages the stomach and digestive organs.

Steps

a) Lie on your back with arms on both sides and legs together but active with toes facing the ceiling.

b) Take a deep breath and as you do so, gently fold your right leg and hug tightly with both hands.

c) As you exhale, draw the leg towards the chest and simultaneously lift your head and upper body so as to touch the knee with your forehead. Stay here for a few seconds, hold on to your breath and engage your bandhas (interior body locks).

d) Inhale as you rest the head back and release the leg on an exhale. Come back to the resting position with arms by your side.

e) Repeat this movement with your left leg.
f) Finally, with the same breath pattern and slow movement, repeat this asana (posture) with both legs.

Benefits

This asana (posture) helps digestion by removing flatulence from the system. This is a good stretch for the femur, inner thigh muscles and the back.

7. Anantasana (Lying Sideways and Leg Lift Pose)

(a)

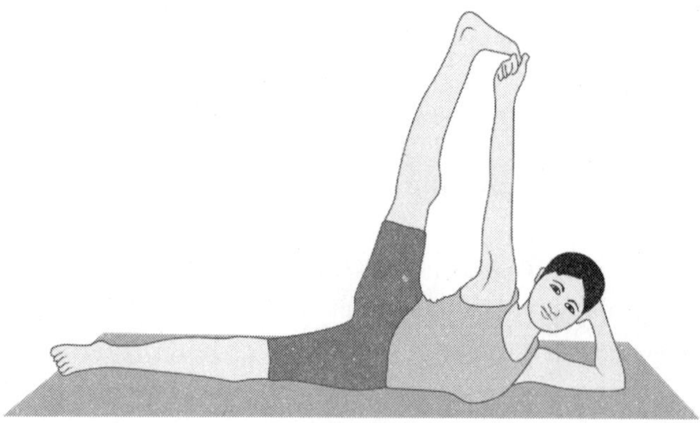

(b)

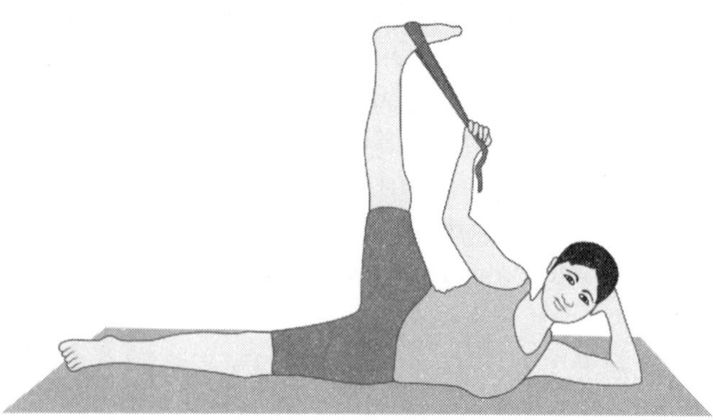

This is a beautiful relaxing asana (posture) and is derived from the resting pose of Lord Vishnu on his abode, the King Cobra (Serpent God Adisesha).

Steps

a) Lie down on your back and turn over to the left side. Extend the left arm over your head and rest the right arm on your right hip. Shift your entire balance on the left rim of your body without tilting forward or backward and define your equilibrium.

b) Once you feel stable, bend the left elbow and support your head with the hand placed just above the ear. Relax your neck muscles and soften your facial expression. Smile.

c) Take a deep breath and slowly bend your right leg at the knee and hold onto the big toe with your right hand. In this position your right knee should face the ceiling and the hips and pelvis should open up.

d) Finally, with an exhalation, raise your right leg high up and straight without releasing your hold of the big toe. Breathe normally.

   Since this is an intense stretch of the legs coupled with balance, you may have to steady yourself first before trying the final posture. Initially you can practice the first three steps and then raise your right leg. If you feel you are unable to hold on to your big toe, you can use a belt or a strap, to loop over the right leg and hold it and then try to stretch the leg. This may be quite challenging for those with tight hamstrings.

   Close your eyes to take a few breaths. Slowly release the hold and bend your leg and come back to step (a) before turning to lie down on your back, in savasana (corpse pose). Repeat on the other side as well.

Benefits

This asana (posture) is meant to make you feel the joy as you close your eyes and visualise Lord Vishnu resting on the King Cobra in the middle of the cosmic ocean. This is supposed to be a meditative pose. At the same time it is intense, as it improves flexibility and stabilises your body. It also stretches the sides of your body, legs, inner thigh, hamstring and waist, and is a great pelvic and hip opener.

However, this posture may cause a stress on the back particularly for those with back problems. They should be very careful whilst trying this asana (posture). The best way would be to rest your back against the wall and use a belt or a rope to hold the legs in position.

8. Naukasana (Boat Pose)

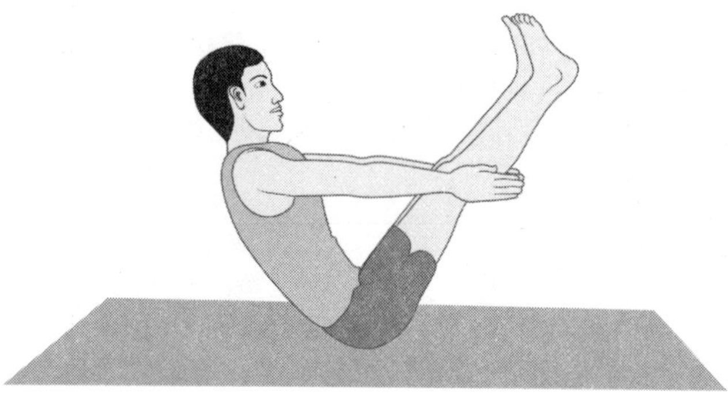

This asana (posture) is a contra pose to any backbend like setu bandhasana (bridge pose) as discussed next or ustrasana (camel pose) which is detailed in the seated series.

Steps

a) Lie down on your back with arms by your side, palms against the body and feet together. Flex your toes and make sure that your leg muscles are firm.

b) Look at the ceiling and take a deep inhalation.

c) As you exhale, engage your uddiyana (abdominal) and mula (root) bandhas (interior body locks) and lift your upper torso and legs simultaneously. At the same time, your arms should also extend forward along with the torso and legs.

d) In this posture you are balancing on your sit bones. It is important to keep your spine and back erect.

e) Fix your drishti (gaze) on the toes or any spot ahead of you. This will help you to find a balance and initially stay in this asana (posture) for a few seconds and with practice for a few minutes. If your gaze wanders, you will find it difficult to balance. Try not to collapse or curve your back. If you do so, the benefits of this posture will dissipate. Initially you might feel the body tremble, but do not worry and try to hold for as long as you can.

   Experienced practitioners will be able to close their eyes and still not lose balance, as their drishti is drawn towards their inner self.

   Take a few breaths and release the posture by coming all the way down to savasana (corpse pose).

Benefits

Naukasana (boat pose) is extremely good for the back and a booster for the abdomen. A terrific posture to strengthen the core and improve concentration, stability and flexibility. The bandhas (interior body locks) also help in conserving and storing energy, leaving you refreshed and rejuvenated.

9. Setu Bandhasana (Bridge Pose)

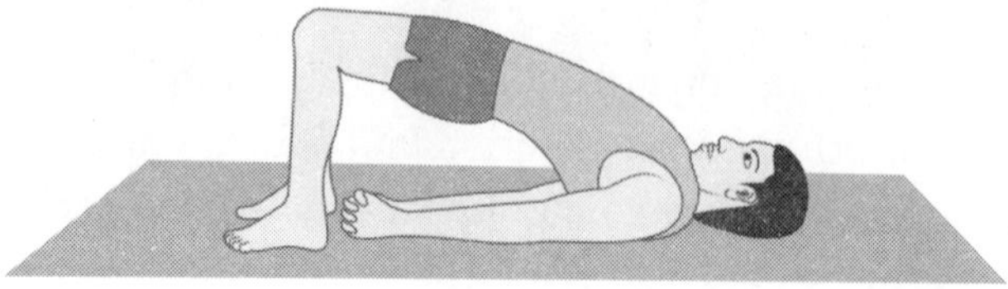

Steps

a) Lie down, bend the knees and draw the legs towards you.

b) Place the feet with toes firm on the floor and arms alongside the body with palms pressed on the floor.

c) Now take a deep inhalation and start raising your chest, lower body and buttocks. Your back will automatically curve and your shoulders and arms will also support the raise. Do not clench the gluteus. Slowly bring arms together and interlock the hands tightly.

Try not to lift your heels in this posture. Initially, you may do so in order to get ready for the body raise. You can also place both hands under your lower back to lift up. But as you sink into the pose your feet should be flat, shoulder blades firm on the floor and hands interlocked.

d) Slowly exhale when you have attained this asana (posture) and strive to lock all your three bandhas (interior body locks).

e) Look towards your chest and relax your facial muscles and neck.

Take a few even, slow breaths and enjoy! In this bridge pose, your chest, belly and thighs should be aligned properly, to form a bridge like appearance.

Release the posture on an exhalation by bringing yourself

down slowly and simultaneously support your back. Bend the knees, draw them towards your chest and embrace with both arms before extending them to relax in savasana (corpse pose).

Benefits

This beautiful half inversion posture stretches and strengthens the back, spine, abdomen, thigh muscles and buttocks. It also stimulates the meridians and connective tissues, thyroid glands, ensures blood circulation and oxygenates the cells in the body.

10. Halasana (Plow Pose)

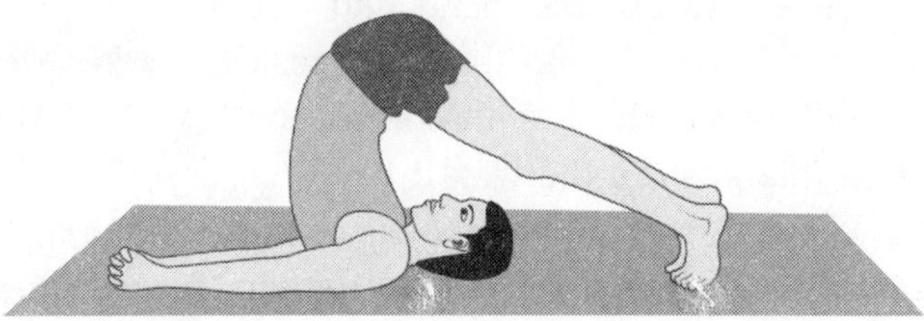

Halasana is a further extension of viparita karani (legs up the wall pose). Halasana can also be attained from paschimottanasana (seated forward bend pose) as explained later.

Steps

a) Follow the steps for viparita karani (as explained earlier) with or without wall support.

b) Take a deep inhalation and as you exhale, allow both suspended legs to gravitate, extend and guide them slowly (avoid a jerking motion) all the way behind till such time that you can feel your spine getting rounded and then straighten with that extreme backbend, until you are able to touch the floor above your head with the tip of your toes. Keep breathing normally.

c) As you do so, support your back with both hands and when you are steady and able to balance, slowly bring both arms close and interlock hands as shown in the illustration. Keep breathing and engage the three bandhas (interior body locks). Stay in this pose for a couple of minutes to reap maximum benefits.

   Take a deep inhalation and release the posture on an exhale with both hands supporting the back and bend your legs to touch the forehead with both knees. Gradually bring your body all the way down to finally relax in savasana (corpse pose).

   This is an intense backbend and you have to be very careful as you get into this posture. Do not rush or be overambitious. Those with core strength will be able to attain this posture the way it has been described above. For women after childbirth, this posture will be extremely challenging almost to the point of saying, "I cannot do it." It is better to attempt easier postures to primarily strengthen the abdominal muscles before trying the plow pose.

Suggestion

Here is a tip for those with a weak abdomen. I learnt this technique when I was unable to extend beyond viparita karani (legs up the wall pose).

Steps

a) Sit erect in dandasana (staff pose). This has been explained in the chapter on seated postures.

b) Take a deep breath and as you exhale bend forward from the hips with arms reaching out to your toes, as in paschimottanasana (seated forward bend pose) which is also explained in the chapter on seated postures. Breathe normally.

c) Take another deep breath and on an exhalation roll backwards with a quick (not jerky) movement lifting both legs, lower body and arms all the way above your head till your toes touch the floor and arms lie above the head, alongside your feet. This forward-to-backward rocking movement helps to roll back easily especially when the abdominal muscles are weak. Adjust the arms and interlock hands.

   Release the posture as explained before.

Benefits

This strengthens your core and conserves body energy since in this asana (posture) you can comfortably lock your bandhas (interior body locks) without much effort. It is a good back stretch and makes the spine strong and supple, improves flexibility and elasticity of the body, and tones leg muscles. It also helps to relax your mind and body and is a calming posture. This asana (posture) is very rejuvenating, you will feel a spring in your movement and instant energy. This posture can also be a precursor to sarvangasana (shoulder stand pose).

11. Matsyasana (Fish Pose)

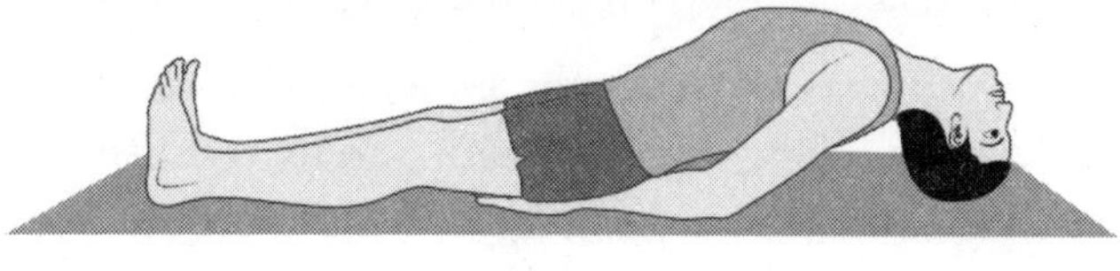

This is a contra pose to inversions. You could do this posture before and after head or shoulder stand pose, as it releases tension in the shoulder joints and neck.

Steps

a) Lie down on your back with feet together.

b) Open up your shoulders and place your hands below your buttocks with palms touching the floor. Your elbows should remain firmly pressed on the floor.

   This can be uncomfortable in the beginning. Make sure you are not wearing any bangle or bracelet, as your attention may get diverted to the discomfort instead of your breath.

c) Deeply inhale, slowly lifting your upper body. Elbows will slightly bend at this stage. Buttocks should be firmly placed on the floor. Please do not strain your gluteus.

d) As you exhale, drop your head to look behind and be very gentle when you do so. Simultaneously flex the feet inwards and feel the full stretch from thigh to calf muscles.

e) Deepen this posture by slightly arching your upper body and slowly let your crown touch the floor, or as close as possible. With practice, some of you may be able to touch the floor with your forehead. Let the body decide your movement.

f) Relax your eye brows, facial muscles and jaws with lips gently pursed. You may tend to open your mouth for comfort. Try not to else you will be breathing through your mouth, which is not correct breathing in yoga practice.

   Close your eyes and relax for a few breaths. Gently release the pose by taking a deep breath and as you exhale, relax your legs and feet and lower your body on the floor and come to savasana (corpse pose).

Benefits

It is a powerful pose for the entire body, releases tension in the neck, opens up the shoulder joints and tones the thighs, hamstrings and calf muscles. It gives a smooth bend for the back and spine and makes them flexible and strong. It also improves blood circulation.

12. Urdhva Dhanurasana (Wheel Pose)

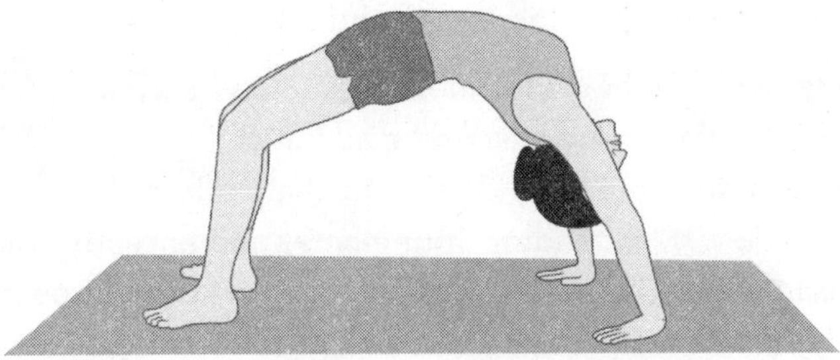

This posture is an intense backbend and needs immense strength in the arms as you have to raise your body and balance on all four limbs in a backward bend. This is also a contra pose to naukasana (boat pose) or halasana (plow pose). Once you are confident and comfortable with setu bandhasana (bridge pose), you can move on with this asana (posture).

Steps

a) Lie on your back and take a few breaths. You need all the energy that you can muster to get into this pose.

b) Take a deep breath and bring both hands close to your ears, elbows bent to face the ceiling and palms on the floor with fingers facing inward, as you take the support of Mother Earth.

c) Exhale and steady yourself in this pose. Bend the legs and place both feet firmly on the floor a few inches away from your buttocks.

d) Now take another deep breath and as you exhale slowly lift your torso. Simultaneously drop the head behind nice and loose such that your crown is just above the floor.

e) Look at the space behind you. Fix your drishti (gaze). Allow your head and neck to hang loose. Keep breathing.

f) Your spine should take a nice C curve and your feet should be firm on the floor. Take a few breaths here.
This is truly an athlete's pose and requires strength in the upper body, spine, abdomen and arms.

Try not to hold on for more than a few seconds to avoid losing balance and sustaining an injury.
Take a deep breath and as you exhale release this posture very slowly by bending your elbows and knees and slowly rest your body on the floor. Draw both knees towards the chest, hug with both arms and rock your body, forward and backward, after this intense abdominal stretch and backbend. Slowly bring both legs down and straighten it with arms alongside to rest in savasana (corpse pose).

Benefits

It has all the benefits of setu bandhasana (bridge pose). This is also a more intense workout and has a deeper impact on your core strength. This posture lends elasticity and flexibility to the back and spine. It stretches the entire spectrum of muscles supporting the frontal body as well as strengthens the arms, wrists, upper thigh muscles and calves. Needless to add, this asana (posture) improves blood circulation and helps to maintain youth by stimulating the facial muscles.

13. Supta Virasana (Reclining Hero Pose)

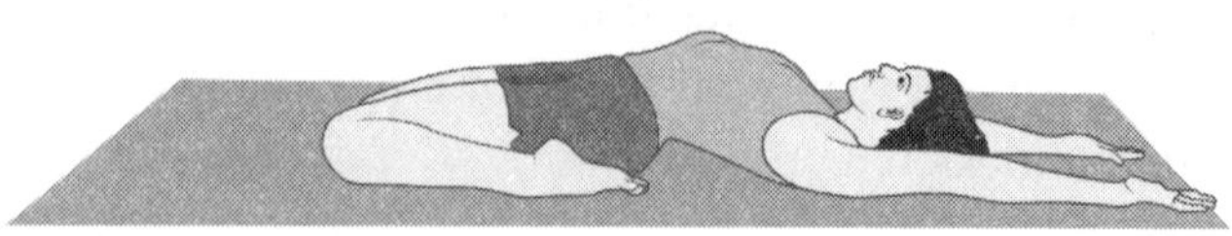

This is a very dynamic and restorative yin posture. This asana (posture) stretches and strengthens the back and thigh muscles.

Steps

a) Sit in virasana (hero pose).

b) Place both hands on your lower back to support it and deeply inhale.

c) As you exhale, lower yourself and take elbow support. Make sure your back is straight and does not hurt.

d) Then slowly lower yourself all the way down with both arms resting on either side, above your head. If your back feels uncomfortably arched, then you may use a pillow for support. Close your eyes, relax and breathe.

   Take a deep breath and on an exhalation release the posture by slowly getting up. Remember to use both hands to support the base of your spine and also take elbow support first before coming back to virasana (hero pose). Relax in balasana (child's pose) to massage your back and to release any tension. This is explained in the chapter on seated postures.

   Alternatively, you may also start this posture from vajrasana (thunderbolt pose). As you lower yourself all the way down, by following the steps explained before you can thereafter adjust the legs with feet to the side or let it remain under your buttocks. Do what works for you without inducing or enduring pain.

Tip

If any asana (posture) causes pain, safely assume you are doing it incorrectly or perhaps overstretching yourself. Listen to your body first and then your body will automatically start listening to you.

Benefits

This is another restorative asana (posture) and has a calming effect on both the mind and the body. It also massages the back and stretches the thigh and abdominal muscles, lubricates knee joints and infuses energy and concentration.

14. Sarvangasana (Shoulder Stand Pose)

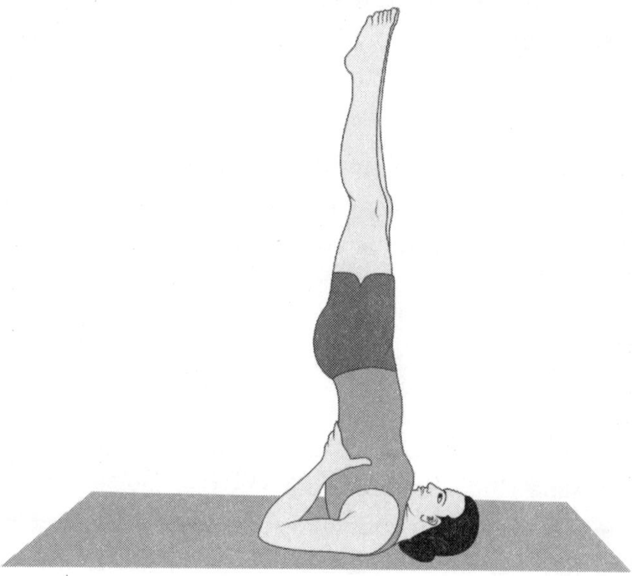

This serene pose, sarvangasana (shoulder stand pose), known as the queen of all asana (postures), is an intense inversion posture and a contra pose to any backbend.

True to its name 'sarva-ang-asana' (entire body parts pose), this posture stimulates all parts of the body. In this asana (posture) the entire body weight rests on the shoulders and upper arms, and rest of the body is suspended in the air as straight as a pole. This should be your ultimate goal as you start practising this posture.

However, in the beginning, you can start with half sarvangasana (half shoulder stand pose), where you may take the liberty to rest a portion of your back on the floor and use wall support for the legs.

It would not be wise to try for the correct pose in the initial stages. You have to be patient and take it in increments and judge for yourself, based on how flexible your body is. Even for those with flexible bodies, there will be days when the body is rigid and stubborn.

Steps

a) Lie down on your back and relax your body.

b) Close your eyes and deeply inhale and exhale a few times.

c) When you are ready, take a deep inhalation and as you exhale, engage your uddiyana bandha (abdominal lock) and bring together both legs with feet touching each other and slowly raise your legs. As you do so, support the upper torso with your hands, to avoid injuring the back.

d) Raise your torso higher up, keep adjusting your hands and tuck in both elbows. Fix your gaze on the navel or chest as you raise the torso.

   In this position, your chin is firmly pressed to your neck or just below it, as if you are testing for a double chin. Thus jalandhara bandha (throat lock) gets automatically activated.

   You are meant to rest only your shoulders, upper arms and head on the floor and the rest of the body must stand tall and elegant in a straight line. Your hands should support your back with the elbows tucked in as shown in the illustration. At this stage it is easy to also lock the mula bandha (root lock).

Keep breathing evenly and look at the toes or close your eyes to enjoy the posture.

Take a deep breath and on an exhalation release the posture slowly by bending both legs simultaneously and bring the knees to your forehead. Then gently lower the back with support of your hands and rest the body on the floor. Thereafter release hands and straighten both legs to relax in savasana (corpse pose).

This is the ultimate posture with all the bandhas (interior body locks) locked for that perfect flow of energy within the body. But to get here, it is alright if you are able to do a half-shoulder stand pose, initially, wherein you rest a tiny portion of your back on the floor. This will help you to achieve the full stance eventually.

Suggestion

A good dose of practice of viparita karani (legs up the wall pose) and halasana (plow pose) will help you in sarvangasana (shoulder stand pose). When you are comfortable with this posture, it can also be another way of attaining halasana (plow pose).

Benefits

It is a perfect balancing posture with energy flowing backwards from mula bandha (root lock) to jalandhara bandha (throat lock). This asana (posture) is an energy booster, stimulates all parts of the body, lifts a few years off your biological age and makes you feel young and raring to go. It also improves concentration, flexibility, stability, body balance, strength and makes you feel wonderful.

I am particularly fond of this posture, although I do tend to use a small slice of my back to balance the torso.

14

Prone Postures

(Lying on the Belly)

This series comprises of the following:

1) Dhanurasana (Bow Pose)
2) Bhujangasana (Cobra Pose)
3) Salabhasana (Locust Pose)
4) Urdhva Mukha Svanasana (Upward Facing Dog Pose)
5) Sphinx and Seal Pose

1. Dhanurasana (Bow Pose)

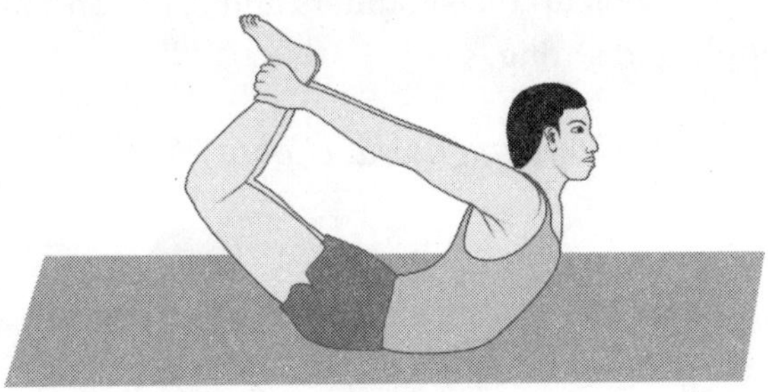

This asana (posture) is an intense backbend and is not too hard to achieve.

Steps

a) Lie down flat on your belly with the forehead resting on the floor and arms alongside with palms facing upwards. Bend both legs and gently hold the ankles with your hands.

Keep the grip firm but not tight.

b) Take a deep breath, raise your upper body and keep bending it backwards. Open up your shoulder joints to make this movement nice and easy. Simultaneously pull the legs inwards and raise the thighs. Try to keep both legs together, but if this is difficult, you may slightly widen them.

c) At the final stage your entire body should be above the floor, except the abdomen and pelvis. Keep breathing.

   Take a deep inhalation and release the posture exhaling slowly and come down on your belly with the face tilted and resting sideways.

Benefits

This asana (posture) has similar benefits as urdhva dhanurasana (wheel pose), except that this is easier to perform and hold. It strengthens the thigh and calf muscles and stretches the entire upper body, opens up the shoulders and chest, and makes the spine supple and strong.

2. Bhujangasana (Cobra Pose)

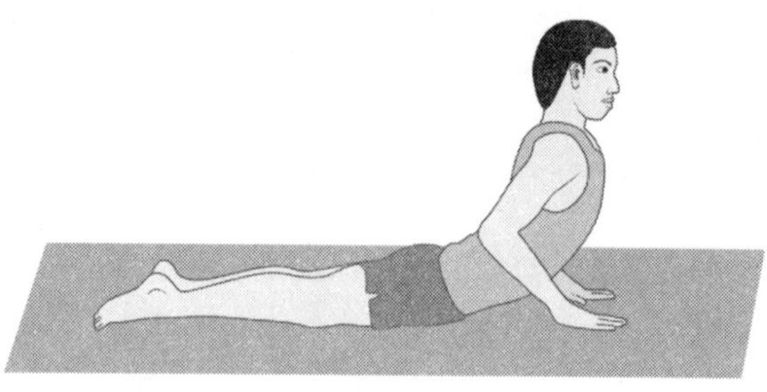

This is a beautiful and subtle backbend and a good exercise for the shoulder joints as well.

Steps

a) Lie down on your belly with both hands pressed on the floor, just below the shoulder joints. Rotate your shoulders to loosen up the joints and feel at ease. The chest will open up automatically. The forehead is to rest on the floor and feet are to be held close together with toes pointing towards the back.

b) Now take a deep inhalation and slowly raise your upper torso. Stomach onwards the entire body should be on the floor. Look straight and fix your drishti (gaze) on any point. As you raise your torso, your hands can also be a few inches above the ground level but in the same position, with elbows bent. Stay here, breathe, enjoy and balance, for a few minutes.

c) Take a deep inhalation, and as you exhale lower all the way down to the floor with head resting sideways and arms on either side.

Benefits

This is a good asana (posture) to strengthen the back as well as the spine. It opens up the chest and releases tension in your shoulder joints and strengthens the arms. This posture also tones the hamstrings, buttocks and calf muscles. Overall, it calms the mind and improves concentration.

3. Salabhasana (Locust Pose)

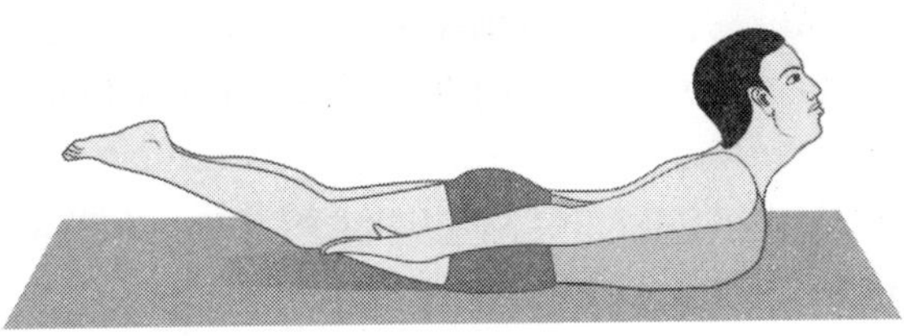

This is one of the most challenging postures although it may appear to be simple. The spine has to be extremely flexible to get this right. Even if you are able to do more than 50% of the legs raise, you should consider it well done.

It is better to start with half-locust position first.

Steps

a) Lie down on your belly with your forehead on the floor. Both arms are to rest on either side with palms facing upwards and fists clenched. Take a deep breath and slowly raise your right leg, without curling the toes of the left leg. You will feel an intense bend of the spine. Bring the foot down as you exhale. Now repeat the same with the left leg.

b) Repeat this twice or thrice, as a warm up for the final locust pose. Relax and take a few breaths.

c) Now open up your shoulders and rotate them in a circular movement. Bring your arms closer to each other as much as possible.

d) Take a few breaths with your forehead on the floor and both arms by the side. With a deep inhalation, lift both legs and arms as shown in the illustration. Consciously relax your gluteus as you will automatically tighten them whilst lifting both legs. Keep the legs together and try not to widen them.

   Hold for a few seconds and then slowly release as you exhale. You will realise that when you raised one leg at a time, you were able to lift it high up. But when you tried lifting both legs, they would have barely been six inches off the floor. That is the challenge of this posture and each body will adapt differently at its own pace.

Suggestion

Initially you could tuck your hands under the thighs, with both palms on the floor. This will act as an impetus for the leg raise, especially when you lift both legs.

Benefits

This is a tough pose and excellent for the back and spine. It tones the leg muscles and releases tension in the shoulder blades.

4. Urdhva Mukha Svanasana (Upward Facing Dog Pose)

This has already been explained in the chapter on surya namaskar (sun salutation) sequence.

5. Sphinx and Seal Pose

(a) Sphinx pose

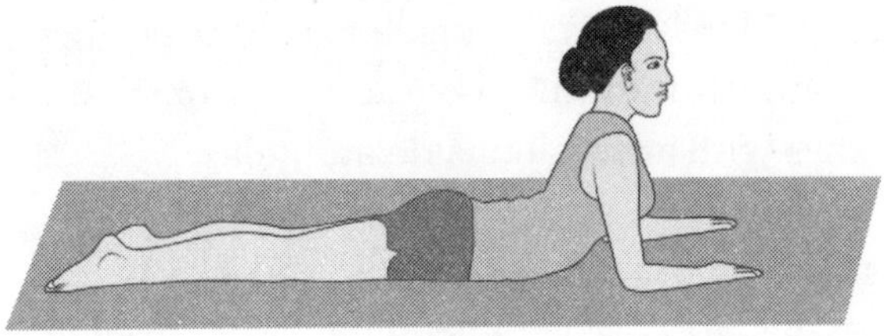

(b) Seal pose

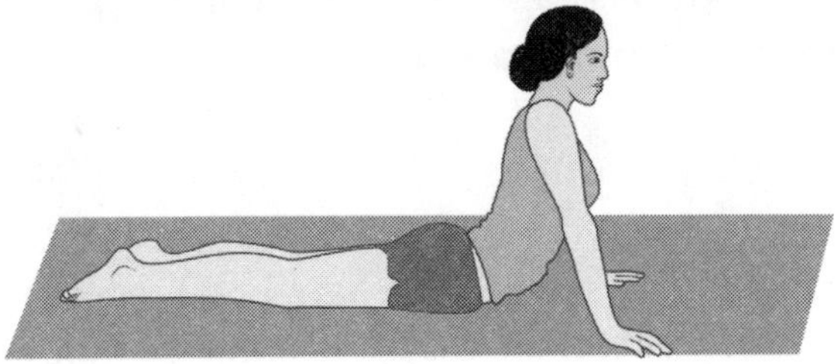

These are restorative postures and typically used in yin yoga.

Steps

a) Lie on your belly and prop yourself up on your elbows as shown in the first illustration.

b) Feet should rest roughly six inches apart.

c) Open up your shoulders. Relax your gluteus. Keep the back erect and look ahead.

d) Relax the neck and facial muscles. Close your eyes and take a few breaths. Enjoy your sphinx pose.

e) Take this a bit further for the seal by lifting the chest straightening the elbows as much as possible. You can bend your elbows slightly if there is too much pressure on your back. The tendency will be to contract your gluteus, but please do not do so. Relax all your body muscles and hold this position and take a few breaths.

   Release the posture after taking a long deep breath and on an exhale slowly lower yourself to sphinx position first and then come all the way down to the floor. Rest your head sideways with arms alongside and relax.

Benefits

Both these postures are very calming and rejuvenating. Apart from strengthening the spine and back, they also help in toning your entire body, massage the stomach and digestive organs and improve concentration and meditation.

15

Seated Postures

The seated postures, also known as the floor series, comprise the following asana (postures) and are fairly simple and excellent to start with especially after completion of the sun salutation sequence.

1) Balasana (Child's Pose)
2) Virasana (Hero Pose)
3) Vajrasana (Thunderbolt Pose)
4) Cat and Cow Movements
5) Dandasana (Staff Pose)
6) Ustrasana (Camel Pose)
7) Gomukhasana (Cow Face Pose)
8) Shoelace Pose
9) Baddha Konasana (Cobbler or Butterfly Pose)
10) Malasana (Garland Pose)
11) Paschimottanasana (Seated Forward Bend Pose)
12) Dragon Pose
13) Tadpole and Frog Pose
14) Bakasana (Crow Pose)
15) Dolphin Pose
16) Pigeon and Sleeping Swan Pose

1. Balasana (Child's Pose)

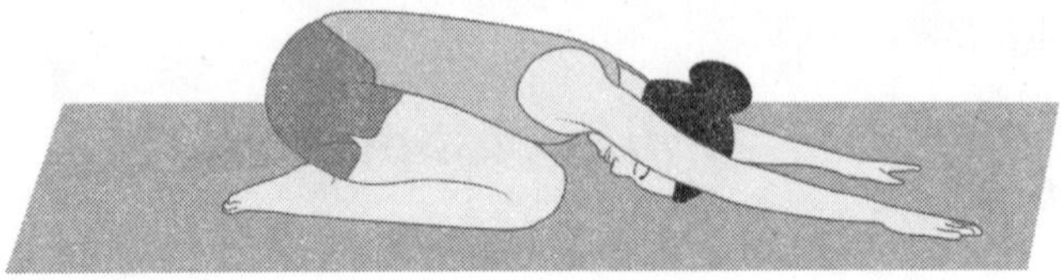

This is a typical relaxation pose and usually the first asana (posture) in a yoga class, after the initial savasana (corpse pose).

Steps

a) Sit with legs folded under your gluteus and knees apart, almost to the width of the yoga mat.

b) Raise your arms above the head, take a deep breath and as you exhale engage your uddiyana bandha (abdominal lock) and extending from the hips, bend forward keeping both arms close to your ears almost brushing it. Shoulder joints should be as close to your ears as possible. Bend all the way down like a seated prostration.

c) Reach out with your arms forward and stretch as much as you can. Please make sure that you do not lift your gluteus. Your sit bones should be where they were at the start of the posture. If you find your body rising, then prop up a tiny cushion below your sit bones.

d) Take a few breaths.

e) In order to make this posture a bit more dynamic, lift your elbows a few inches away from the floor and shift the balance of your hands on your fingertips, inhale and reach forward by few millimetres as you exhale. Keep doing this till you have reached the maximum point. Breathe softly and enjoy.

Take a deep inhalation and when exhaling, release this posture and sit in virasana (hero pose) or vajrasana (thunderbolt pose) with both hands on your thighs and palms facing upwards.

Benefits

This asana (posture) stretches the upper torso admirably and is a great spine and abdomen stretch. It also tones your arms, releases any tension in the shoulder blades, relaxes your facial muscles and adds colour to your cheeks.

2. Virasana (Hero Pose)

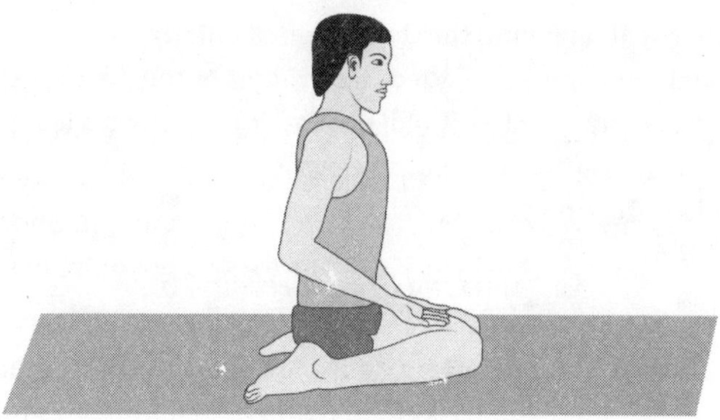

This is one of the basic seated postures and well-suited for pranayama (breathing exercises). This posture is also ideal for meditation after you have derived comfort in it.

Steps

a) Sit down with knees bent, inner thighs close to each other and tuck the lower part of your legs under the thighs, with feet apart to create just enough space for you to settle down.

b) Keep back and spine erect, and do not slouch.

c) Open up your shoulders and rest both hands on the thighs

with palms facing upwards.

d) Close your eyes or fix your drishti (gaze) on a spot before you and breathe.

Release the posture by stretching your legs and wiggling your toes to improve blood circulation, in case you feel pins and needles.

Benefits

This improves posture, concentration and stability, and stretches your thigh muscles. This is a very restful asana (posture) and can be held for a long time. You can try this asana (posture) whilst watching TV and reap health benefits together with enjoying the daily dose of entertainment. For the spiritual or religious minded, this is one of the good postures that can be practised as it will enable you to sit for a few hours in satsang (prayer) or ceremonies where you are required to be seated on the floor.

3. Vajrasana (Thunderbolt Pose)

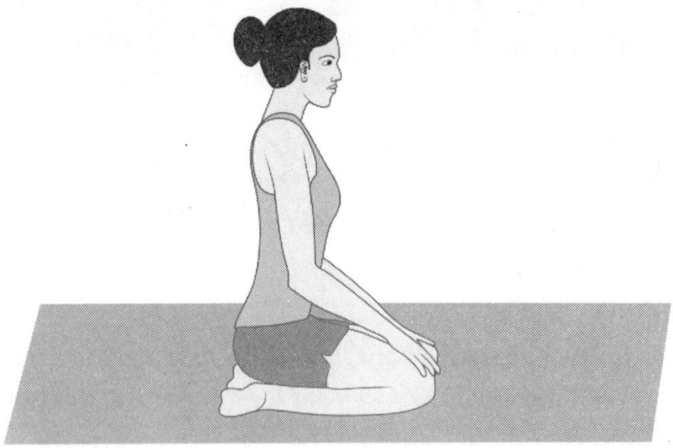

There is not much difference between virasana (hero pose) and vajrasana (thunderbolt pose), except that in this asana (posture) you have to keep the feet together and rest your sit bones on the heels. You do not create space as in virasana (hero pose).

The steps and benefits are similar to virasana (hero pose) and hence are not explained separately here. This posture is also to be released in the manner stated above.

Vajrasana (thunderbolt pose) is popular amongst Japanese particularly in their tea ceremony. It reinforces the fact that this posture can comfortably be held for two to three hours at a stretch.

4. Cat and Cow Movements

(a) Cat

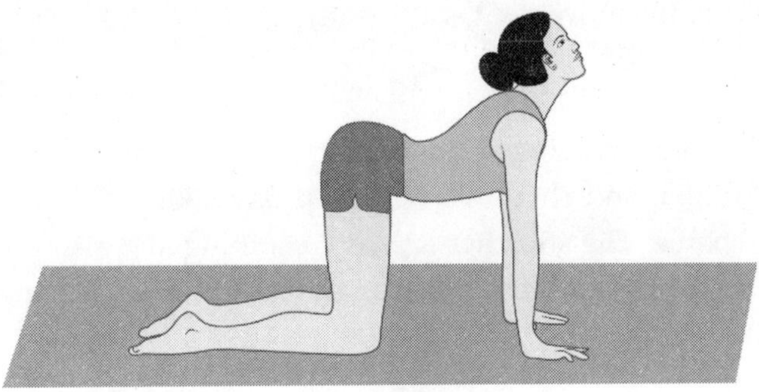

(b) Cow

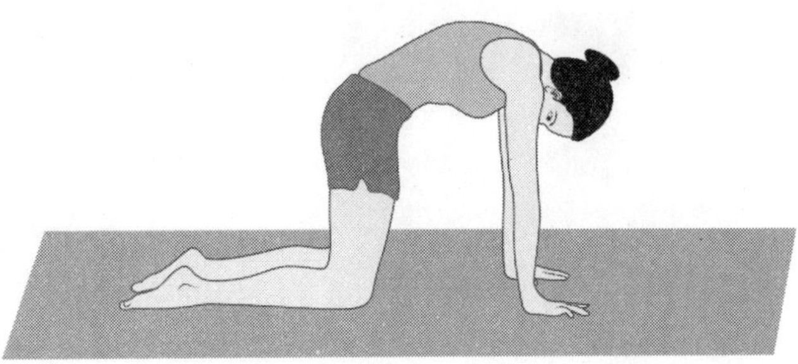

This is a warm up asana (posture).

Steps

a) Come down on both hands and knees. Take care that the hands are placed just below the shoulders and at shoulder width. Legs are to be at hip distance. Align your body well before you start the movements.

b) As you inhale arch your back and look up without straining the neck or facial muscles. Keep them loose and supple. This is your cat as illustrated in (a).

c) Exhale and arch your back and spine inwards as if to round your body. This is your cow as illustrated in (b).

Keep doing this a few times and also draw an imaginative number 8 so as to curve the sides of the body, both ways. Relax the movement and breathe gently.

Benefits

This posture massages the abdomen, back and spine in a comfortable and rhythmic motion thus making it more agile and flexible. The stretches are very soothing and also prepare your body for adho mukha svanasana (downward facing dog pose).

5. Dandasana (Staff Pose)

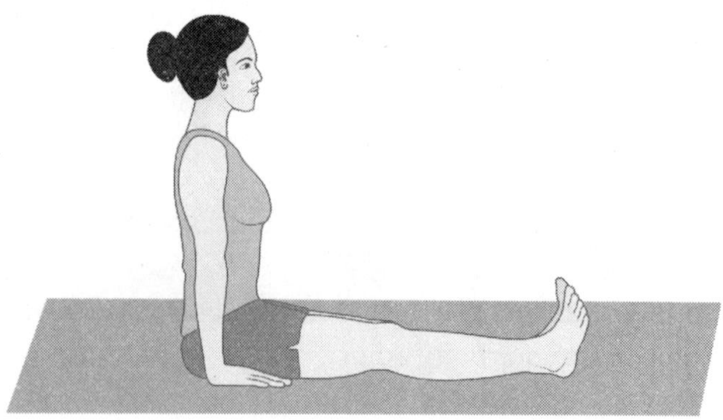

This is an active seated posture and, as suggested by the name itself, this posture has to be held as taut as a stick or staff.

Steps

a) Sit cross-legged and focus on keeping the back and spine very erect. You could use wall support or prop a cushion under your sit bones. But gradually let go of the props and try to sit erect on the mat.

b) Extend the legs and flex your toes inwards, outwards and then inwards. You should feel the stretch in your hamstrings and calf muscles.

c) Open up your chest and rotate the shoulder blades and, with palms touching the floor, take a deep inhalation and lift your body into a more erect position. Make sure your palms are pressed firmly and fingers face the front side.

d) Engage your bandhas (interior body locks) and breathe evenly. Fix your gaze and focus on your breath. Soften your facial muscles and smile.

   Release the posture by relaxing your body and hugging knees against your chest.

Benefits

This is a lovely asana (posture) to improve stance, style, concentration. This asana (posture) is good for the entire back and spine. It also tones your leg and arm muscles and strengthens the shoulders and wrists. The abdominal lock and breathing pattern helps in calming your senses. Maximum benefit is derived in this posture if you are able to let go of the props and achieve this asana (posture) the way it is. At best, wall support can be taken. This is not hard but do give yourself some time to let your body adjust.

6. Ustrasana (Camel Pose)

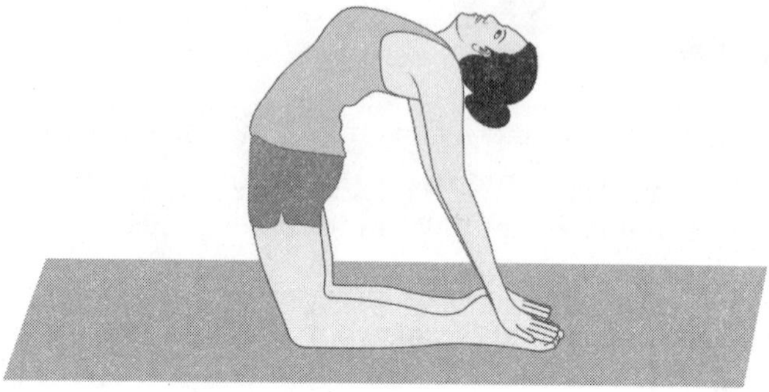

This is an intense backbend and care should be taken to support your back, while getting into the pose as well as coming out of it.

Steps

a) Kneel down. Knees should be at hip width distance and arms by your side. Look straight.

b) Place both hands firmly on your lower back for support.

c) Take a deep breath, as you look up and start the backward bend (in stages) on a slow exhale.

   1st stage: Run your gaze along the ceiling and look halfway behind and bend slightly.

   2nd stage: Bend all the way behind, as much as you can, with the neck hanging loose. Please do not strain your neck muscles. Fix your drishti (gaze) on the space behind you.

d) Simultaneously release both hands and rest your palms on the sole of the feet. Alternatively, you may grip both ankles during the initial stages of practice.

   Breathe here in this position, although you may find it hard to swallow the saliva. Please do not hold your breath however tempting it might be. Release the position slowly and as you exhale, come back to the kneeling down position, by supporting your lower back as before. Settle into balasana (child's pose) to soothe your back and relax.

Suggestion

If you are unable to reach your feet or ankles, you could try curling your toes to rest palms on the heels. Alternatively, you may place two wooden blocks by your side and rest your hands on them. No matter how you do it, this intense backbend is a good contra pose for all the forward folds, regardless of the option you may choose.

Benefits

This posture makes your spine very strong, flexible and supple and also stretches the upper torso – chest, abdomen and pelvic region. It releases tension in the neck muscles, shoulders and upper back, oxygenates your body and improves blood circulation. It also strengthens your shoulders, thigh muscles and legs. This posture will make you feel young and vibrant.

7. Gomukhasana (Cow Face Pose)

(a)

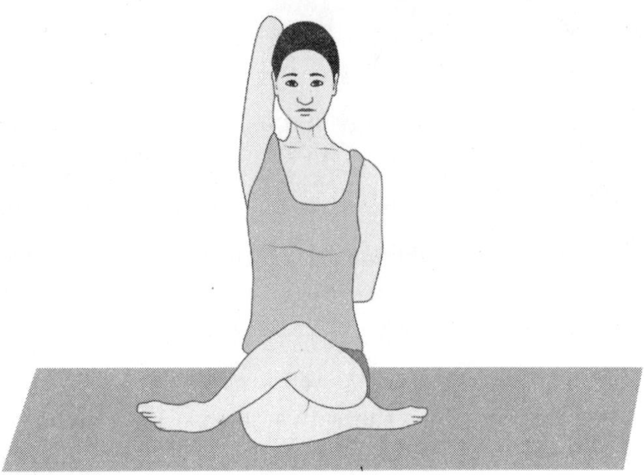

(b)

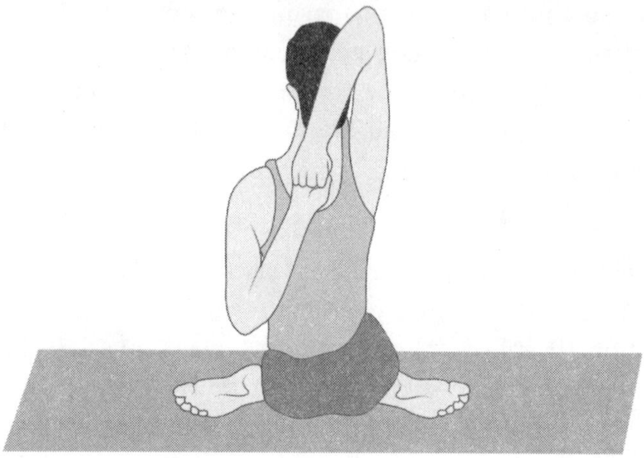

This asana (posture) is a dynamic pull and stretch resistance workout of the upper body.

Steps

a) Start the posture by getting down on both hands and knees. Interlace your legs by placing the back of your left thigh over the right thigh.

b) Slowly sit down on the floor without releasing your grip. You may use a cushion under the buttocks to support your sit bones.

c) Take a deep breath and loosen your shoulder joints and open up your chest and shoulders.

d) Raise your right arm above your head and reach upwards by extending it from the shoulders. Keep stretching and relax your joints.

e) Take your left hand behind and rest it on your upper back. Keep opening up your shoulders so that your left arms can extend as high as possible.

f) Now bend your right arm and interlock your hands. Hold it with a firm grip as shown in illustration (b).

Look straight and freeze your drishti (gaze). Relax your neck and facial muscles. Smile and breathe. Hold for a while and release the posture by freeing your hands. Gently release the legs and wiggle your toes.

Benefits

This is perfect resistance training due to the pull and stretch motion. It strengthens your arm and leg muscles particularly the triceps, biceps, quadriceps and shoulder joints. The intense upper body stretch improves posture, concentration and stamina. This is also an excellent stretch for the spine.

Eye Rotation Movements

When you are comfortably seated and settled in gomukhasana (cow face pose), start the eye rotation. This helps in strengthening your eye muscles.

1) Imagine a gigantic clock ahead of you.

2) Keep your head straight and steady. Look up and slowly rotate your eyes clockwise.

3) At every number pause for a second, till you arrive at to where you began.

4) Repeat this in an anticlockwise direction.

Rub your hands, cup them and cover both eyes. This is

very soothing especially when your eyes are puffy and tired. Repeat this a few times.

These eye exercises can also be practised seated in vajrasana (thunderbolt pose), if you wish. However it helps better in gomukhasana (cow face pose) as your head remains steady because of the intensity of the upper torso stretch.

8. Shoelace Pose

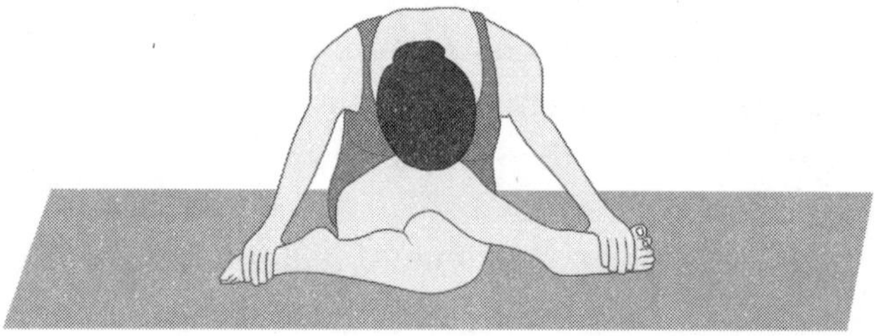

This is one of the yin postures which can be held comfortably for two to three minutes. It is a modified version of gomukhasana (cow face pose), without the resistance pull and stretch element. This asana (posture) is more restful with the main focus on flexibility of the spine and back and relaxation.

Steps

(a) & (b) are the same as explained under the cow face pose.

c) Take a deep breath, open your chest and slowly bend forward by extending from your hips. Bend as much as your body permits.

d) If you are able to rest the forehead on your knee, as show in the illustration, that would be a good start.

e) Then slowly attempt to bring the chin on your knee with the head above the floor.

f) The ultimate position is to bring your crown to the floor, as the elasticity of your spine improves and your back becomes more flexible.

Benefits

This restorative posture helps in overall relaxation of your mind and body. It also massages the digestive organs and stomach, relaxes the back and increases flexibility, apart from making the spine supple. This posture tones your facial muscles by improving blood circulation.

9. Baddha Konasana (Cobbler or Butterfly Pose)

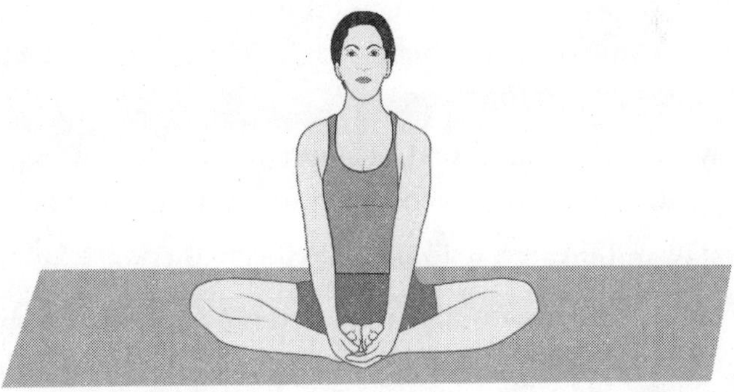

This is a lovely pose and can turn into an intense forward bend if you desire. This is a yin posture, as well.

Steps

a) Sit down erect in dandasana (staff pose). Prop up a light cushion to support your sit bone, so that you are comfortably seated. You could use wall support initially to keep your spine and back straight.

b) Bend your knees and draw feet together towards your groin, so that the soles of your feet touch each other.

c) Keep rocking your knees and try to press it to the floor. This may be uncomfortable initially but you will surprise yourself at the comfort you will feel in this position with some amount of practice.

Those who wish to take this further into a yin posture can follow these steps:

d) Take a deep inhalation, tuck your abdomen, lock it and on an exhale, slowly start the forward bend by holding your feet with both hands to propel forward. Your elbows will automatically take the support of your inner thighs. Activate the root lock.

e) Let go of the hold and take another deep breath and come forward all the way down, on an exhale, till such point where your body stretches to the maximum. Extend the arms to rest on the floor.

f) Try to lock your throat, jalandhara bandha, by pressing chin just below the hollow of your neck.

g) Relax and take a few breaths.

Take a deep breath and release the posture on an exhale by slowly coming up and stretch your legs and wiggle the toes, to get back the blood circulation.

Suggestion

Try not to slouch or arch your back in this asana (posture). When your knees touch the floor you will feel an intense stretch in your inner thighs and groins. In case your leg hurts, place two cushions or pillows on either side so as to rest your knees.

Benefits

It is an intense stretch for your inner thighs and a hip/groin opener as well. It is good for the spine and back as it increases flexibility. This posture improves blood circulation and concentration. Engaging the body locks helps in removing energy blockages and creates a sense of calmness and balance in both the mind and the body.

10. Malasana (Garland Pose)

(a)

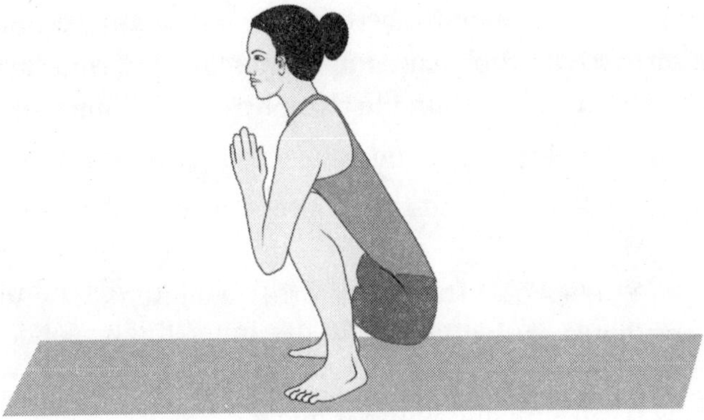

(b)

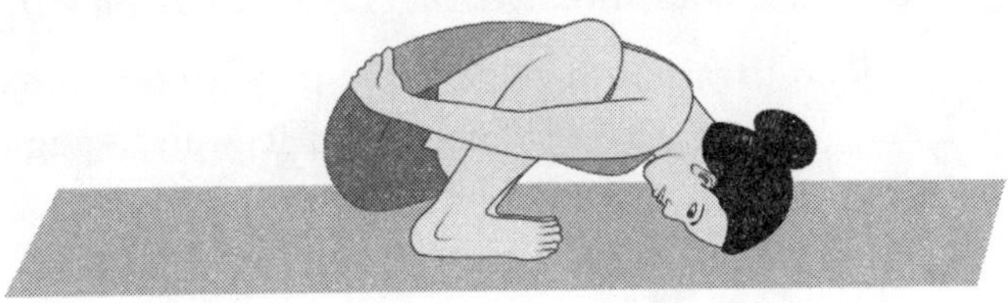

This is the squatting posture.

Steps

a) Stand with feet hip distance apart. Extend upper body forward from the hips, in a halfway lift position from the floor with hands on the knees. Take a deep breath and slowly come down to the squat position, on an exhale.

b) Keep the spine straight and bring hands in prayer position. Place your forehead on the finger tips and relax. How simple it is!

Those who want to make it more dynamic may follow the below-mentioned variation.

c) Bring your feet closer, take a deep breath and on an exhale bend forward as much as you can, and touch the floor with your forehead as shown in the illustration.

d) Hug your back with both arms and clasp the hands. Alternatively you may simply stretch the arms forward and rest your hands on the floor. Keep breathing normally.

Complicated? It is actually fun trying it, so do check this out!

Benefits

This asana (posture) opens up the hips and groins, lubricates the knee joints and strengthens the inner thigh, pelvic and abdominal muscles. This is also one of the yin postures in which you can sink into without much effort.

11. Paschimottanasana (Seated Forward Bend Pose)

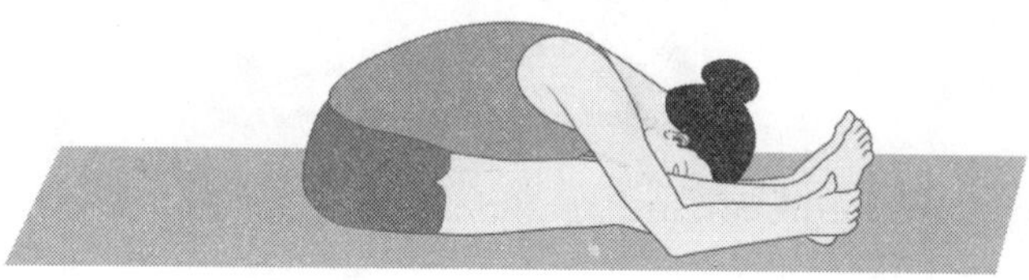

This is a contra posture to backbends like dhanurasana, the bow pose.

Steps

a) Sit in dandasana (staff pose). Keep a cushion under your sit bone, to be able to sit tall with the spine erect. Look straight ahead.

b) Take a deep breath and raise both arms above your head and hold them close to your ears; it would be even better if you are able to bring the shoulders closer to your ears. As you exhale lengthen from the hips and bend forward. Lock the abdomen (uddiyana bandha). Whilst taking the bend, bring your arms down with the upper torso, without altering the position. This puts an added pressure on your abdomen and helps in strengthening it.

c) Try to hold your toes with both hands. Bring your head down to rest on your thighs. Keep breathing.

d) For those who have been able to do the above, hold your feet with both hands, take another deep breath and upon an exhale extend a bit further to bring the forehead on or below your knee.

   Keep breathing and release the posture with an exhalation, by raising your body and arms together and come back to the staff pose. Rest hands on your knees or on the floor and relax.

Suggestion

Please do not fret if you are unable to touch your toes. You can use the belt and loop it over your toes and hold it firmly with both hands and then bend forward as explained above.

Benefits

This posture is a superb forward bend, good for the spine, abdominal and leg muscles. It has similar benefits as halasana (plow pose). This is also a powerhouse posture for storing your energy by locking all the three bandhas (interior body locks) simultaneously.

12. Dragon Pose

(a)

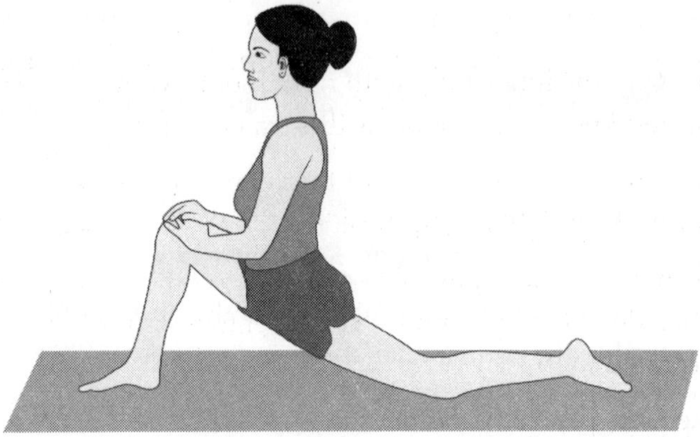

(b)

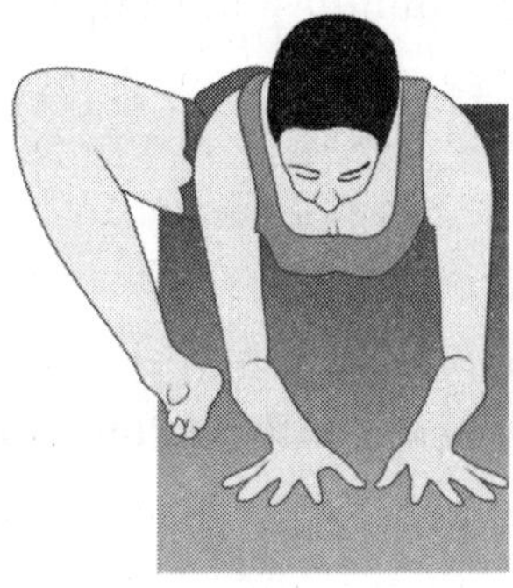

(c)

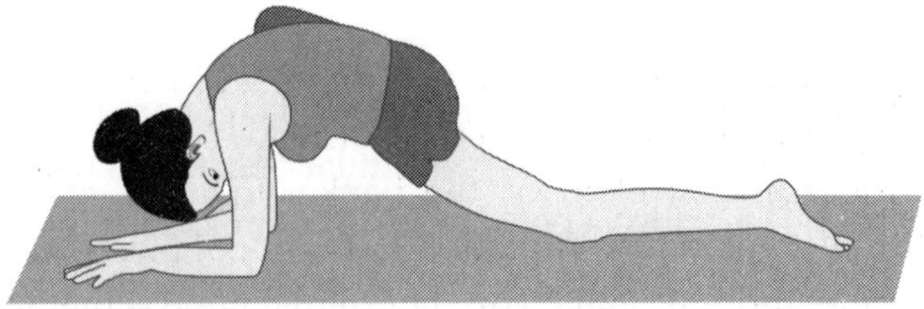

This is one of the most uncomfortable yin postures, nevertheless excellent for toning, stretching and opening up the body. This posture is more towards taking the lunge to the next level.

Steps

a) Start with the lunge pose with right foot forward and bring your left knee on the floor, as illustrated in (a).

b) Place your hands on the right thigh and look ahead. Keep your back straight and spine erect.

c) Slowly inch your right foot towards the outer edge of the right side of the mat and tilt your feet to rest on the rim, as illustrated in (b).

d) Take a deep breath and on an exhale, lean forward to rest your elbows and bend down as illustrated in (c).

   Stay here for a few minutes and take deep breaths. You will want to release the posture as soon as you settle in it. I do understand that this is quite an uncomfortable asana (posture). But it is worth making an effort to hold this lovely yin posture so as to reap its benefits.

   Slowly come up on an exhale and release the posture back to lunge position. Repeat with the left foot.

   Release and come down on your hands and knees before settling down in vajrasana (thunderbolt pose).

Benefits

This is a deep stretch for the inner thighs and leg muscles in particular and a great hip-to-groin opener. This is a perfect toner and stretch for the back and increases the flexibility of your body. This terrific body balance pose is also calming and will make you feel rejuvenated when you come out of it.

13. Tadpole and Frog Pose

(a) Tadpole Pose

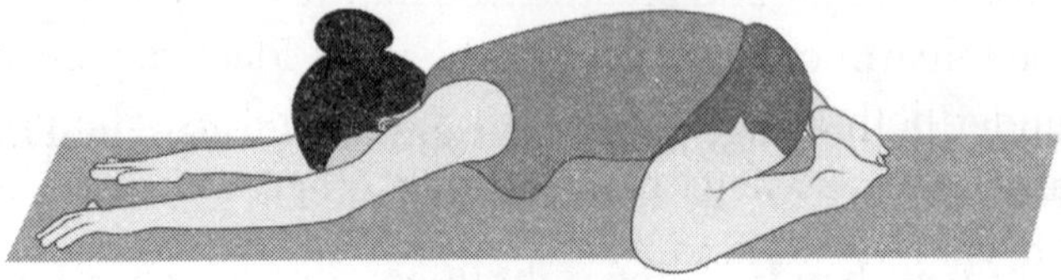

(b) Frog Pose

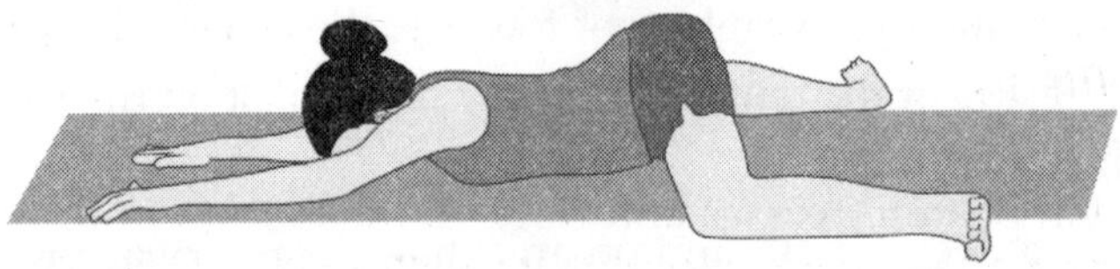

This is yet another yin posture and an amazing hip and pelvic opener. It also deeply stretches the inner part of your thighs and is a lovely back stretch.

Steps

a) Kneel down with both knees wide apart. Take a deep inhalation.

b) On an exhale, lock the uddiyana bandha (abdominal lock) and slowly come forward on your elbows and then lie down on the floor with sit bones raised and toes touching each other, as shown in illustration (a). Keep both arms outstretched above the head and rest your forehead on the mat. This is the tadpole pose where you can engage the body locks. Keep breathing.

c) Take another deep breath, release the toes and widen the gap between the two legs, lift your hip with the tailbone raised higher as shown in illustration (b).

d) Your stomach, pelvis and thighs will be on or marginally

above the floor in this stance. Your toes will face outwards.

Hang on to this position of 'comfortable discomfort' and close your eyes and breathe. You may rest your forehead on the forearm or the pillow or the floor. Place tiny cushions under both knees, if required. Gently release the posture and bring the legs close to each other and come down on your hands and knees. A few cat and cow stretches will help to massage the back before sitting in vajrasana (thunderbolt pose).

Benefits

This yin posture relaxes and releases the tension in the lower part of your body by opening up your hips, groin, abdomen and pelvis. It massages your inner thighs. It also makes your hips and lower back very supple and stretches the upper body magnificently. This yin posture helps to improve blood circulation and concentration.

14. Bakasana (Crow Pose)

(a) Crow Pose

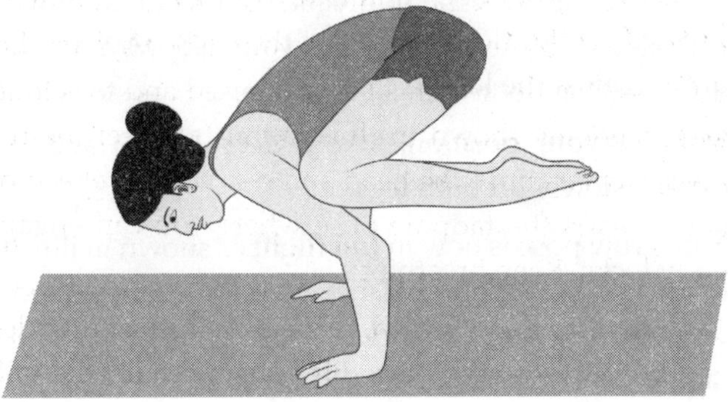

(b) Baby Crow Pose

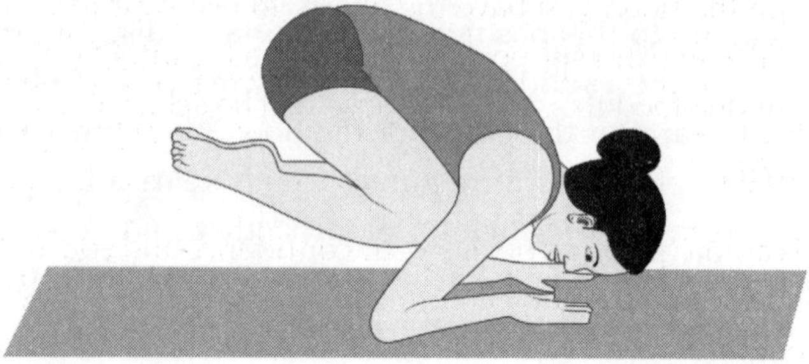

This is a perfect posture for strengthening the biceps, triceps and quadriceps. It is a fantastic body balancing posture. This is also a very dynamic and powerful asana (posture), hence not done in a yin class.

Steps

a) Start with step (a) of malasana (garland pose).

b) Focus your drishti (gaze) on the floor and position your upper arms to rest on the inner part of your knees and raise the heels.

c) Press your hands firmly on the floor and place your body weight on your arms without straining the wrist.

d) Gently rock your body and take full support of your hands pressed on the floor as well as the support of your upper arms against the knees.

e) Stabilise your position, take a deep breath and, as you exhale, slowly lift both legs.

   Your crow pose is now in full flight as shown in illustration (a). If you are able to balance here for a few seconds, you deserve a pat on your back. Release gently and stand up in tadasana (mountain pose) and breathe.

   Baby crow as illustrated in (b) is for those who need moral encouragement before attempting the crow pose. The stance is almost the same except that instead of pressing the hands on the floor, you have the liberty to use your forearms and take an extra support to practise the leg lift. Once you have understood this, the crow pose will be achievable.

Benefits

This asana (posture) boosts your confidence and concentration. It is a great balancing posture and an acid test to determine the strength of your arm muscles and wrists. It is a challenging asana (posture) that also strengthens the abdominal muscles, builds stamina and conserves energy.

15. Dolphin Pose

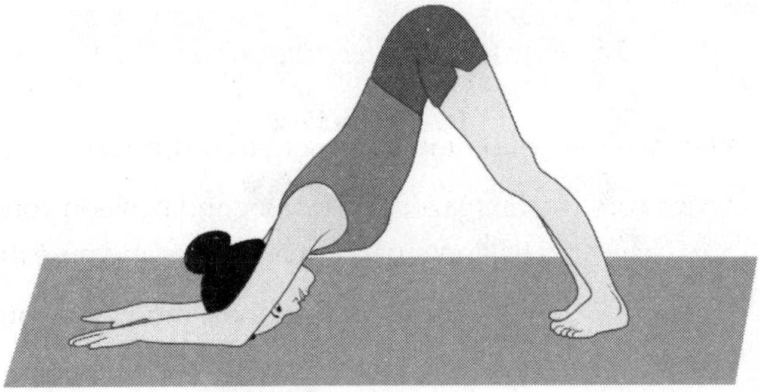

This is a sweet inversion posture.

Steps

The technique is similar to downward facing dog pose except in this posture, you are meant to place your forearms on the floor for support and bring the crown to rest in-between both elbows, and then lift your whole body up with the tailbone tilting upwards. Press the feet firmly on the floor. Those with tight hamstrings may slightly bend the knees. Follow the same breathing pattern as explained under the downward facing dog pose.

Release the posture when ready and come down on hands and knees and sit up in vajrasana (thunderbolt pose) and relax.

Benefits

All the advantages of an inversion posture can be derived in this asana (posture). It also strengthens your calf and thigh muscles in addition to the spine and back. Locking the bandhas (interior body locks) will direct proper energy flow and make you feel happy. This posture improves body balance, concentration and memory. The facial muscles become relaxed with enhanced blood circulation and supply of fresh oxygen to your cells. This lovely posture will help you to achieve sirsasana (head stand pose) comfortably.

16. Pigeon and Sleeping Swan Pose

(a) Pigeon Pose

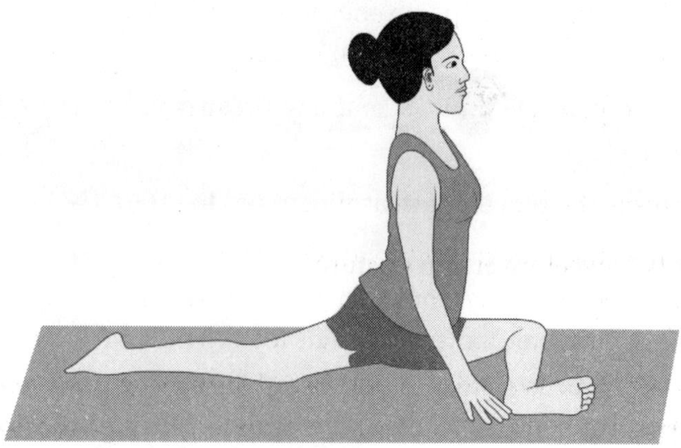

(b) Sleeping Swan Pose

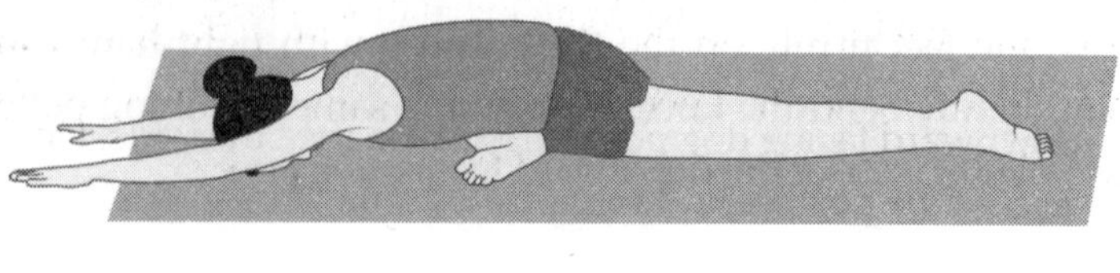

This is another beautiful and restorative yin posture. It is a lovely hip opener and an upper torso stretch.

Steps

a) Start from adho mukha svanasana (downward facing dog pose).

b) Lift the left leg behind long and straight and as high as you can with a deep inhalation, similar to the downward facing dog pose with a leg raise.

c) Exhale, bend the knees and place the left foot close to the little finger of your right hand, and sit down.

d) Stretch the right foot backwards and position it on the centre of the mat. Rest your arms on either side. You will feel an intense back stretch. Keep your spine straight. This is very important.

e) Rest your fingertips on the floor and look ahead without straining your neck or facial muscles.

f) Close your eyes and take a few breaths. Do not curl your toes.

   This is the pigeon pose as illustrated in (a).

g) Take another deep breath, elongate the spine and on an exhale slowly come all the way down. Engage your uddiyana bandha (abdominal lock) in this position. Rest your forehead on the floor and extend your arms forwards.

   Close your eyes and breathe freely. You are now in the sleeping swan pose, as illustrated in (b).

   Take a deep breath and on an exhalation release the posture and come down on hands and knees and get into the downward facing dog pose to repeat on the other side. Finally release the posture and relax in savasana (corpse pose).

Benefits

This posture is very soothing for the back and spine. It also massages the digestive organs. The elongation and stretch will make you feel very fresh and calm both in the posture as well as when you come out of it.

16

Standing Postures

In this chapter, I have explained various balancing postures that enable stability and body balance.

God forbid! But in case you happen to have an accidental fall, there are good chances that you might escape without breaking any bones if you diligently practice these asana (postures). Subconsciously your body will take the impact in the right manner and in hindsight you will realise that yoga practice was a lifesaver.

This tip is neither a figment of my imagination nor an exaggeration, but based on my own experience. I have had two consecutive falls on snowy days in one of those wintry mornings in New Zealand. I must have walked very fast without estimating the ice hidden beneath the snowflakes which could flip you off the ground. Undoubtedly, my body did hurt a bit due to the impact, but I was in one piece and able to get on with my day.

When I was narrating this incident to my friends in the yoga class, my instructor heard it and remarked that practising the standing series had held me in good stead. I noted this in my diary that night.

The various balancing asana (postures) are as follows:

1) Tadasana (Mountain Pose)
2) Adho Mukha Svanasana (Downward Facing Dog Pose) with leg raise

3) Utkatasana (Chair Pose)
4) Parivrtta Utkatasana (Twisted Chair Pose)
5) Virabhadrasana 1,2,3 (Warrior Pose 1,2,3)
6) Viparita Virabhadrasana (Reverse Warrior Pose)
7) Parsvottanasana (Intense Side Stretch Pose)
8) Prasarita Padottanasana (Wide Legged Forward Bend Pose)
9) Trikonasana (Triangle Pose)
10) Parivrtta Trikonasana (Revolved Triangle Pose)
11) Utthita Parsvakonasana (Extended Side Angle Pose)
12) Parivrtta Parsvakonasana (Revolved Side Angle Pose)
13) Padahastasana (Forward Bend with Hands under the Feet Pose)
14) Padangushtasana (Forward Bend and Toe Hold Pose)
15) Urdhva Prasarita Eka Padasana (Standing Splits Pose)
16) Natarajasana (Dancer Pose)
17) Vriksasana (Tree Pose)
18) Ardha Chandrasana (Half-moon Pose)
19) Vasisthasana (Side Plank Pose)
20) Garudasana (Eagle Pose)
21) Sirsasana (Head Stand Pose)

1. Tadasana (Mountain Pose)

This asana (posture) has been explained and illustrated under the surya namaskar (sun salutation) series and hence the explanation is not repeated here.

2. Adho Mukha Svanasana (Downward Facing Dog Pose) with Leg Raise

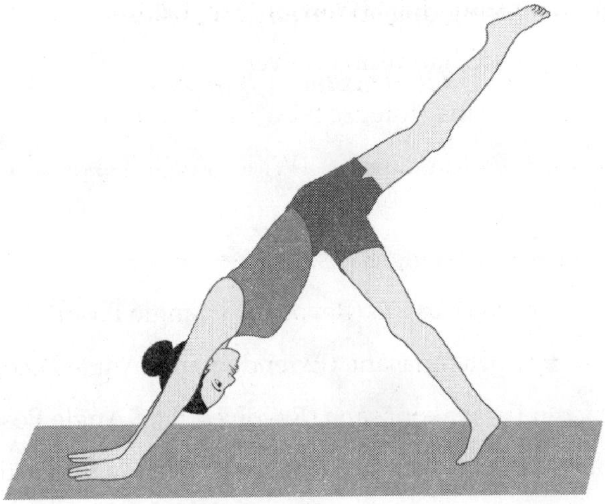

Adho Mukha Svanasana (the downward facing dog pose) has also been explained in the sun salutation series. Here I have suggested a slight variation to this with leg raise which is a fantastic hip and groin opener.

Steps

a) Take the position of downward facing dog.

b) With a deep inhalation lift your right leg.

c) Your shoulder, spine, back and leg should be well-aligned.

d) Exhale, bend the knee and bring the right leg forward to touch your forehead with the knee. Repeat the above actions once more time.

   Repeat on the other side. Release the position and come down on your hands and knees and sit in vajrasana (thunderbolt pose).

Benefits

A great hip and groin opener, this has similar benefits as stated in downward facing dog and inversion postures.

3. Utkatasana (Chair Pose)

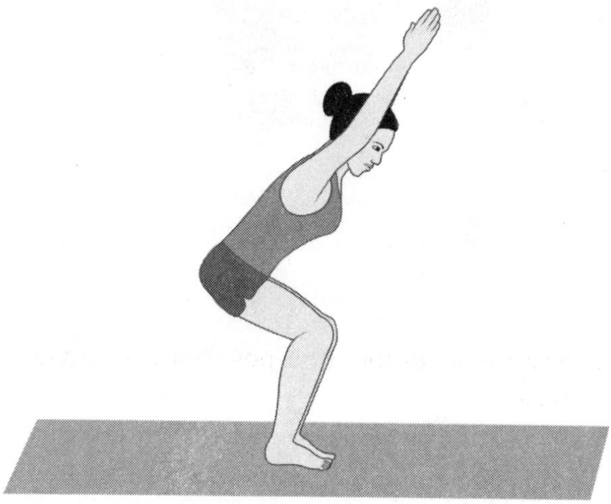

This is the imaginary chair pose.

Steps

a) From tadasana (mountain pose) take a deep inhale and raise both arms over your head alongside your ears. You must feel a deep stretch from the shoulder joints.

b) Place your feet close to each other and with a deep exhalation, sit down as much as you can. Keep back and spine erect.

Benefits

This asana (posture) tones and shapes up your thighs, calves and gluteus. It also helps you to balance in an awkward position thus challenging your stance, builds stamina and improves concentration.

4. Parivrtta Utkatasana (Twisted Chair Pose)

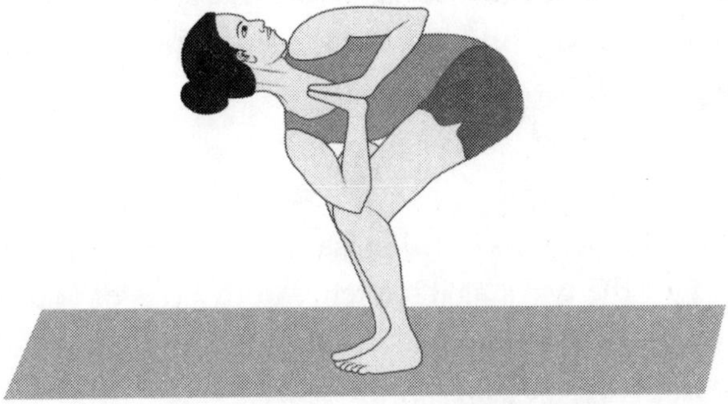

This asana (posture) takes the chair pose to the next level with a bend and twist.

Steps

a) From utkatasana (chair pose) take a deep inhalation and with hands in anjali (prayer position), gently bend forward from the hips elongating your spine, as you exhale. Take care to not get up from the imaginary chair. You may feel your legs tremble initially but later it will get steady.

b) Take another deep breath and on an exhale twist to your left placing your right elbow over your left leg to propel you to twist further. The right elbow can rest above your knee or left thigh, depending on how much you are able to twist. Look up. If you wish, you can release your hands, left hand upwards and right hand to touch the floor. Remember to twist from your waist. Keep breathing and hold onto this position.

c) Take a deep inhalation and release this posture with a deep exhalation and come back to the centre still seated in utkatasana (chair pose). Repeat the twist on the right side, in the same manner.

With a deep breath release the asana (posture) on an exhalation and stand up in tadasana (mountain pose) to relax.

Benefits

Apart from the benefits of utkatasana (chair pose), the twist is very good for the waist as it stretches both sides of your upper body, hips and the spine, making it more strong and flexible. This also improves stability of the body.

5. Virabhadrasana 1, 2, 3 (Warrior pose 1, 2, 3)

(1)

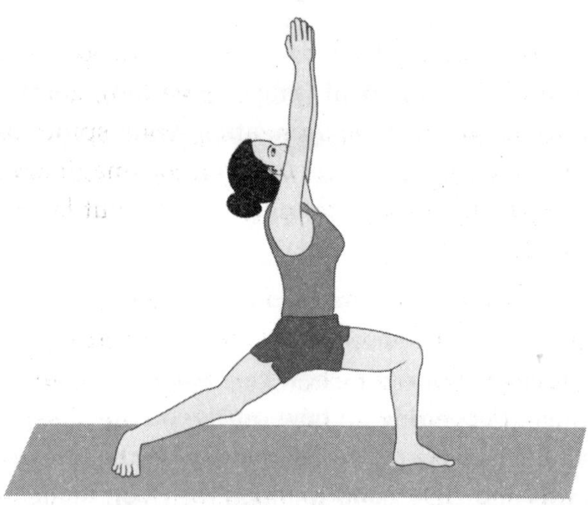

(2)

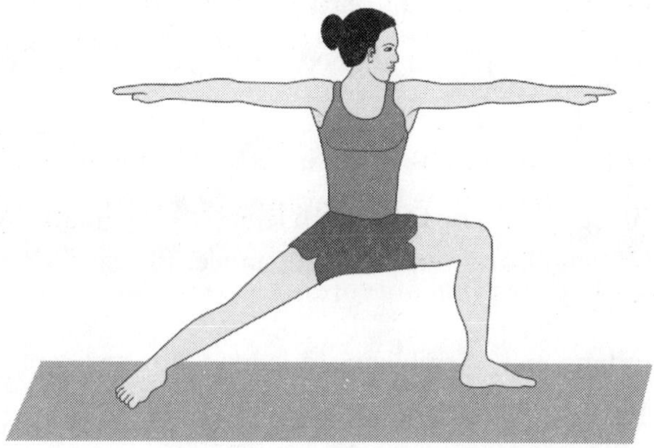

(3)

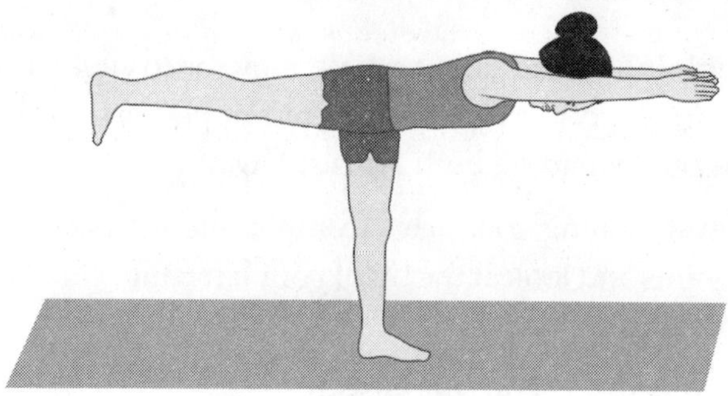

The Warrior pose is a very robust and powerful asana (posture) with many variations designed to exercise the legs and the lower body intensely.

Steps

Virabhadrasana 1 (Warrior pose 1):

a) From tadasana (mountain pose), extend your left leg forward or bring the right leg backward and place both feet firmly on the floor. Inhale deeply and bend the left knee on an exhale. The knee should be in line with your ankles and not the toes. Many of us tend to make this mistake initially.

b) Your thigh should be aligned with your hips and parallel to the floor.

c) The left leg should be in an 'inverted L' shape.

d) Right leg should be firm. Both legs should equally take the body weight and support the stance. Please do not raise the heel.

e) Simultaneously, arms should extend upwards and palms should be joined lightly as in anjali (prayer pose).

   Look up and lock your gaze. Breathe normally.

Virabhadrasana 2 (Warrior pose 2):

a) Deeply inhale and as you exhale, move on to virabhadrasana 2 (warrior pose 2) by twisting your upper torso to the right side and extending both arms sideways.

b) Keep stretching your arms from the shoulders, and loosen the joints and look at the tip of your left hand. Take a couple of breaths in this pose.

Virabhadrasana 3 (Warrior pose 3):

a) Deeply inhale and as you exhale, take the position of virabhadrasana 3 (warrior pose 3) by facing the front and placing your body weight on your left foot, and extend forward from your hips.

b) Your right leg will be on the floor with the heel raised. Steady yourself and fix your gaze on the floor.

c) Now take a deep breath and as you exhale lift your right leg completely off the floor such that it becomes parallel to the floor. Simultaneously extend forward both arms along with your torso. You may join hands in prayer position or keep both arms parallel to each other. Your body stands suspended like a horizontal stick supported by one leg as shown in the illustration 5(3).

Please ensure that your drishti (gaze) does not waver. A steady gaze will help you stay rooted in your posture. Breathe. Release the posture on an exhale, gracefully by placing your right leg on the floor and come to tadasana (mountain pose).

Repeat the three variations of warrior pose on the other side.

Benefits

This asana (posture) improves concentration and body balance. It strengthens the backbone, lower back and legs and releases tension in the shoulder joints. True to its name, this warrior pose enhances your gait and boosts self-confidence.

6. *Viparita Virabhadrasana (Reverse Warrior Pose)*

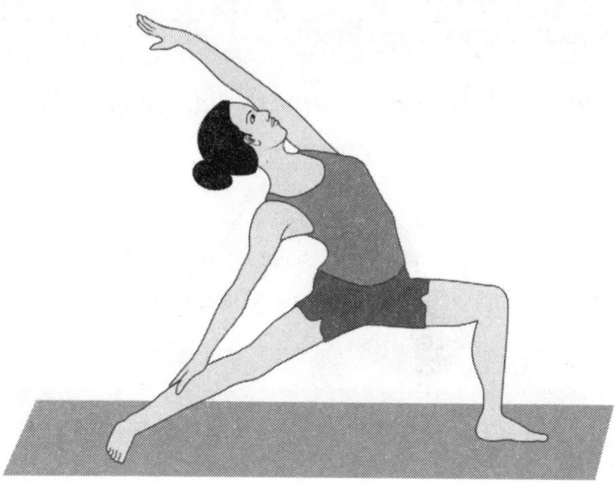

This asana (posture) can be done after Warrior pose 2, before you start the balancing posture in Warrior pose 3.

Steps

a) From warrior pose 2 take a deep breath and, on an exhalation, extend sideways to the right by bending your upper body from the waist, left arm over your head as in an arc and right hand touching your calf, as shown in the illustration.

b) You will feel a deep stretch on the entire left side of your torso as you balance in this posture.

Take a few breaths here. After deeply inhaling, as you exhale gently, release the posture and come back to warrior pose 2 and then relax in tadasana (mountain pose). Repeat on the other side in the same manner.

Benefits

This is an excellent body toner with a deep and satisfying stretch that will invigorate and relax your abdominal and pelvic muscles. It opens up the hips, groin, vertebrae and also strengthens the arms, legs, thighs and calf muscles.

7. Parsvottanasana (Intense Side Stretch Pose)

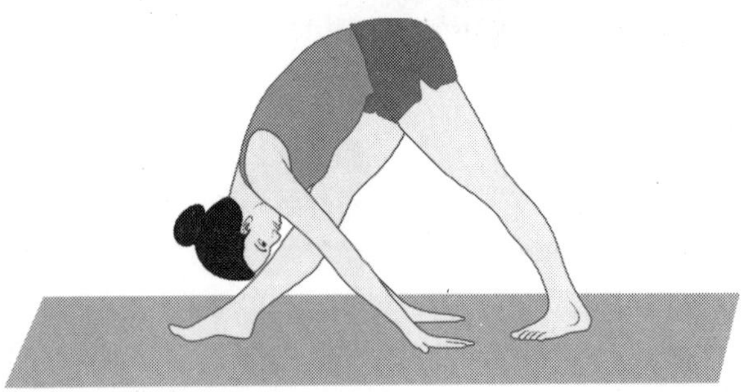

This is an inversion posture with an intense stretch and forward bend.

Steps

a) From tadasana (mountain pose) take your left leg backward with feet positioned at 45 degrees angle as shown in the illustration.

b) Take a deep breath and, as you exhale lengthen the spine, extending forward from your hips and push the right hip backwards such that the upper torso is parallel to the floor. Stabilise yourself and place both hands on the hips.

c) Take another deep inhalation and on an exhale come all the way down such that your forehead touches the knee or below as shown in the illustration. Rest both hands on the floor between the legs. Activate the body locks.

   Please do not force the bend. Do as much as your body permits you to. This sort of an intense bend needs a very flexible body and supple spine. You can use blocks on either side to rest the hands or hold the ankle. Breathe and enjoy the asana(posture). Release on an exhalation and come back to tadasana (mountain pose).

Benefits

This is an extremely intense pose for strengthening the backbone, abdomen and leg muscles, particularly the quadriceps and hamstrings. This asana (posture) has all the benefits of an inversion pose. It oxygenates your body and makes you feel fresh and happy. It improves focus and adds sparkle to your features.

8. Prasarita Padottanasana (Wide Legged Forward Bend Pose)

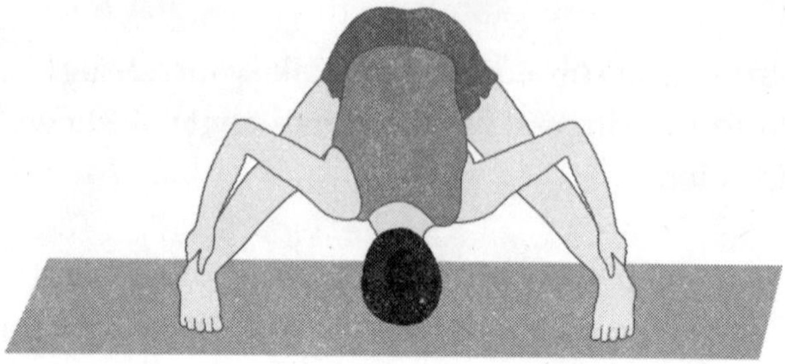

This is another inversion posture and an intense forward bend.

Steps

a) Stand with legs wide apart and do not bend your knees. Fan your toes and keep them firm with the heels rooted to the floor. The upper body should be held erect and the drishti (gaze) steady and arms stretched sideways.

b) Take a deep breath and raise both arms above your head. Remember to always extend from the shoulders to release the tension.

c) As you exhale, engage the abdominal lock and extending from the hips slowly come forward all the way down and try to touch the floor with your crown, if you can.

d) Having done so, place your palms on the floor or hold onto both ankles to freely enjoy this asana (posture). The neck should be totally relaxed to avoid stiffness or pain.

   More experienced practitioners bring their head in line with the two legs. This requires oodles of practice and a very obedient spine. But please do not worry if you are unable to do so. Initially, aim to bring your head as close to the floor as possible. Even this could be challenging for beginners. Please remember to not force the bend and hurt your back. As the body gets more flexible the bend will become easier.

Close your eyes and let go by focussing on your breath. You will be able to lock all the three bandhas (interior body locks) in this asana (posture). After a few breaths, gently open your eyes and take a deep inhalation.

Release the posture as you exhale. Slowly come to the standing position, and then take a bend backwards and finally rest in tadasana (mountain pose).

Benefits

This posture improves circulation of blood, oxygenates the cells, stimulates the abdominal muscles, opens up the hips and groins, enables elasticity of spine and strengthens your back and leg muscles. This has all the benefits of an inversion posture and is a tremendous energy booster.

9. Trikonasana (Triangle Pose)

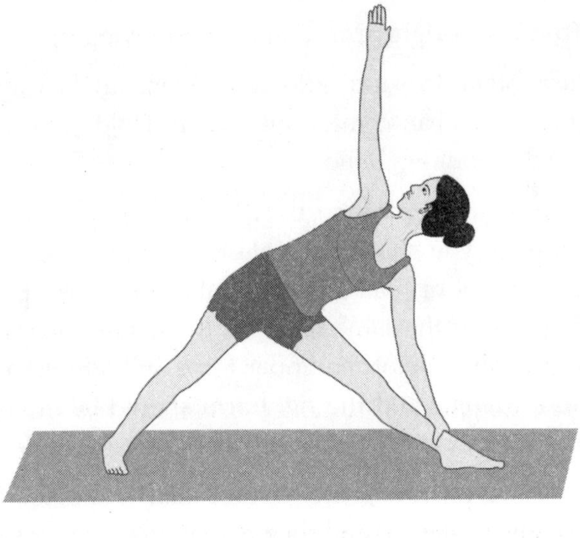

This asana (posture) is an intense sideways stretch and one of the best asana (posture) that can be included in your daily yoga practice.

Steps

a) Start from tadasana (mountain pose) and with a swift jump extend both legs apart – more than your shoulder width but not as wide as in prasarita padottanasana (wide legged forward bend pose).

b) Keep both legs firm. Your toes should lightly grip the yoga mat. Stay rooted. Find your balance.

c) Stretch both arms sideways by extending them from your shoulders as if trying to reach out to both ends. Keep the elbows straight.

d) Keep your back and spine erect and look ahead.

e) Turn your left foot to face the left side.

f) Now deeply inhale and start extending sideways to your left, as you exhale.

   Take another deep inhalation and extend a little more with an exhalation. Make sure your body does not start sagging in front. Your right arm should start moving upwards.

g) Take another deep inhalation and extend all the way down, as far as you can comfortably reach. Hold your ankle or shin with your left hand.

   If you are unable to do so, use a block to support the stance. Eventually you should be able to touch the floor behind your left foot or hold your left ankle and look up to your right hand at the same time. As the name suggests, your left arm, left side of the upper torso and left leg ought to form a triangle and the right arm should be in line with your left arm, for that perfect trikonasana (triangle pose).

   Release the posture gently on an exhale and in increments and come to step (a) and then repeat on the other side.

Benefits

This asana (posture) is an intense upper body sideways stretch and opens up your shoulders, chest and hip joints. It also strengthens the legs and stabilises your body. It flushes out toxins and purifies the digestive system and stimulates the major meridians of your body.

Suggestion

This asana (posture) is difficult to achieve and will take time before you are able to bend sideways from the waist. The tendency will be to collapse forward whilst trying to grip the ankle. This is incorrect and may not help you to reap the benefits of this asana (posture). Therefore, in the initial stages, use wall support and follow the steps. At each stage of bending, feel the wall brushing your back. If not, then you have collapsed in front and need to correct the stance.

Use a block and reaching the block could be your next milestone. Take it slowly and in stages; as your body gets more flexible, you will be able to bend sideways just as you are able to bend in a forward fold.

10. Parivrtta Trikonasana (Revolved Triangle Pose)

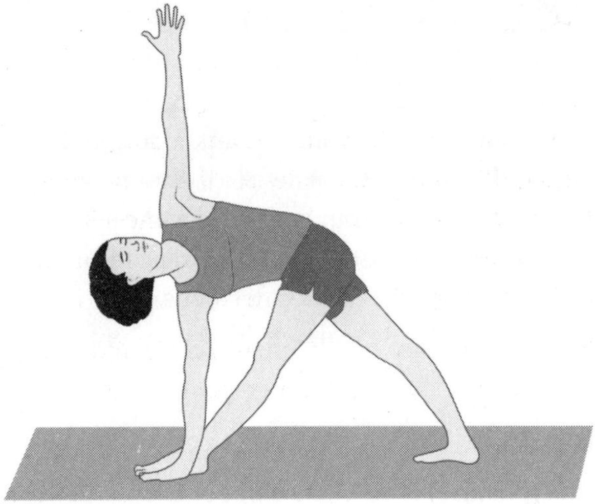

This is a more challenging asana (posture) as it involves a waist twist along with the sideways bend.

Steps

a) Initial steps (a) to (e) are the same as trikonasana (triangle pose) until you are ready to twist, extend and bend.

b) Thereafter twist from your waist to face the left side. At this stage both hands can be on your hips. Keep your knees and feet firmly rooted on the floor.

c) Take a deep inhalation and, as you exhale, twist further to face the back side and slowly bend down. The right side of your body will extend and come down as shown in the illustration.

d) Both arms should be released and extended on either side from the shoulders, to form a triangle with the left leg, right side of the upper torso and right arm as depicted. Align your left arm such that it is in line with your right arm.

   Look up to your left hand and breathe. Release gently on an exhalation. Repeat on the other side.

Benefits

Most of the benefits are similar to that of trikonasana (triangle pose) except that the intense twist of this posture will also increase the flexibility of your waist and make it more agile and slim. It will shave off the excess fat alongside the waist. This is a perfect asana (posture) for improving your concentration and stability. This posture also makes your entire body very supple, especially your spine.

Suggestion

The hardest part is to master the twist and learn to bend

sideways from the waist rather than from the front of the body. A block and the wall will be of immense help to get started on this posture.

11. Utthita Parsvakonasana (Extended Side Angle Pose)

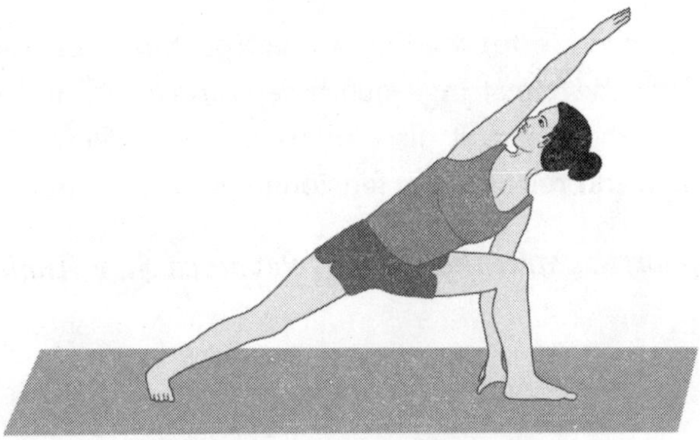

This asana (posture) is another lovely side stretch and all these sorts of sideways bends are a good exercise for your waist, hips, spine and back and makes them more flexible over time. It thus helps in attaining postures like trikonasana (triangle pose) and the twisted postures eventually, even without props and supports.

Steps

a) This asana (posture) is an extension from virabhadrasana 2 (warrior pose 2). Take a deep breath and on an exhale bend your left leg, in such a way that the knee is aligned to the ankle. The left thigh should be parallel to the floor, like an inverted L.

b) Place your left hand near the left foot and extend your right arm above your head onto the left side. You will feel a deep stretch alongside your right waist and hips.

c) Look up and breathe.

Release the posture on an exhalation by slowly standing up in virabhadrasana 2 (warrior pose 2). Repeat on the other side and then come back to tadasana (mountain pose) and relax.

Benefits

This is a wonderful toning asana (posture) for the legs, particularly the hamstrings, quadriceps and calves and a lovely stretch for the waist. It also opens up your chest, shoulder joints, hips and releases any tension in your neck muscles.

12. Parivrtta Parsvakonasana (Revolved Side Angle Pose)

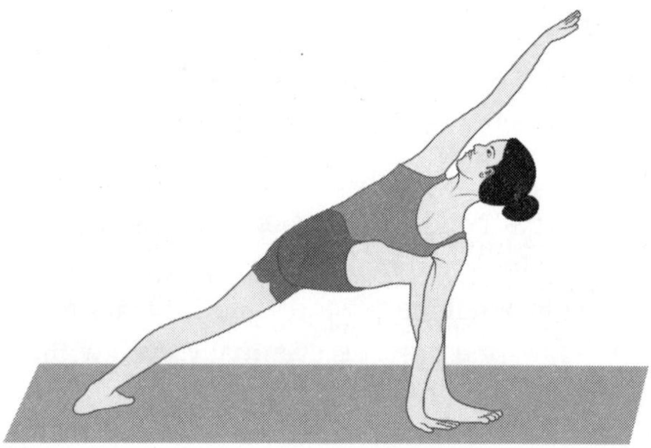

This posture is more intense as it involves a twist of the waist and spine coupled with a sideways extension.

Steps

a) Get into utthita parsvakonasana (extended side angle pose) on your right side. Make sure the alignment is as described earlier.

b) Take a deep inhalation, twist your waist gently and rest your left arm on your right thigh on an exhale. The right arm can be held behind the back for support and to open up the chest. This will also facilitate the twist.

c) Take another deep inhalation and, as you exhale, bring your left shoulder joint to graze your right knee and using this as a support try to touch the floor with your left hand. You may use a block and hold it with your left hand. The right arm is to extend sideways above your head.

   Try to look up or fix your gaze in a convenient spot and breathe.

   Take a deep inhalation and as you exhale slowly release the posture by coming out of the twist first and then to virabhadrasana 2 (warrior pose 2).

   Repeat on the other side. Release and finally come to tadasana (mountain pose) and relax.

Benefits

This asana (posture) increases the flexibility of your spine, back and waist by stretching the upper body on both sides and strengthens your thighs, knees and calves. It also improves concentration and body balance.

13. Padahastasana (Forward Bend with Hands under the Feet Pose)

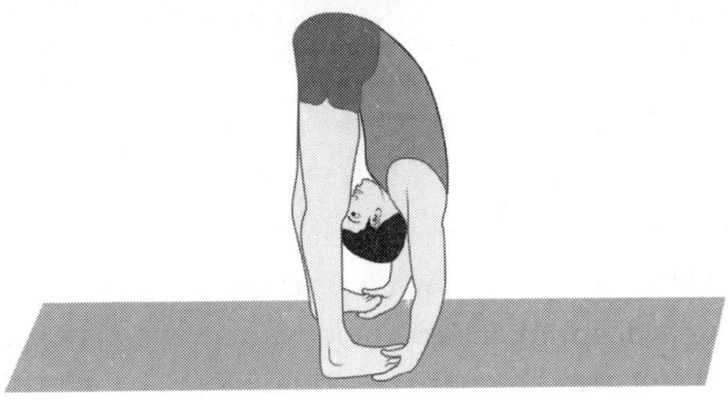

This forward bend is similar to uttanasana (forward bend pose) as described in the surya namaskar (sun salutation) series, but with variation at the end.

Steps

Initial steps are the same as uttanasana (forward bend pose) and hence they are not explained here. The variation starts now:

a) Balance your body evenly on both feet and bring the hands under the balls of your feet. Those with tight hamstrings can slightly bend their knees but as minimal as you need to.

b) Bring the head close to your legs, as if to touch the knee with your forehead with the crown facing the floor. The upper and lower torso should look as if sandwiched or stuck to each other.

c) Remember to engage the uddiyana bandha (abdominal lock) in this forward fold. As you hold the pose you can easily lock the mula bandha (root lock) and jalandhara bandha (throat lock).

   Breathe and enjoy in this inversion posture.

   Take a deep breath and, on an exhalation, release gently by slowly bringing your body up first and then the head all the way up and bend backwards with hands supporting the back, to ease the spine. Come back to tadasana (mountain pose) and relax.

Benefits

This pose stretches and strengthens the prominent muscles in the body, stimulates the meridians improves body balance and sharpens the memory; coupled with all the other benefits of an inversion posture.

14. Padangushtasana (Forward Bend and Toe Hold Pose)

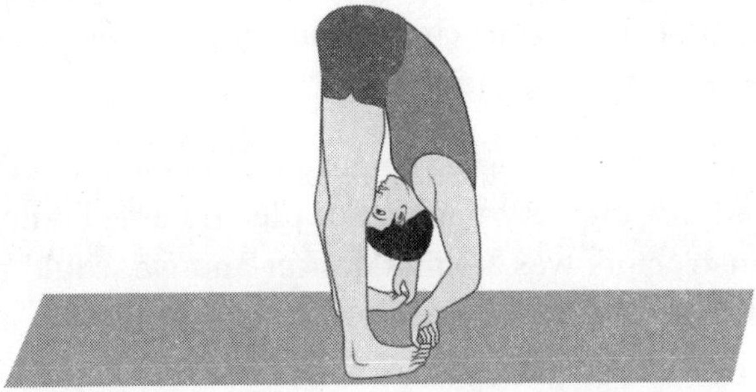

This is yet another variation of the above-mentioned asana (posture). The slight difference being that here you hold the big toe and balance. This is a bit easier to balance than the previous posture, as your toes are on the floor and the weight of your body can be held with ease. The steps and benefits are similar, hence these are not explained here separately.

15. Urdhva Prasarita Eka Padasana (Standing Splits Pose)

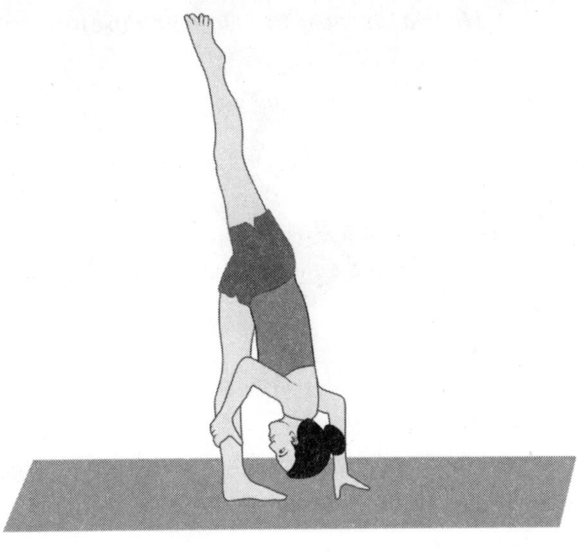

This posture is an extreme variation of the above two forward bends. This can best be attained from virabhadrasana 3 (warrior pose 3) or ardha chandrasana (half-moon pose), with wall support for the leg raise.

It is extremely challenging to get this alignment and splits are meant for the very young, supple and able bodies. One of my instructors was a ballet dancer and we would merely watch her do the splits, attempting was a dream to most of us.

Benefits

This is a hip and groin opener apart from having all the benefits of an inversion posture. It is recommended for the super flexible bodies. It stretches the inner thigh muscles and is also a spine stretch and massages internal organs of the body. It improves blood circulation and makes you feel rejuvenated.

16. Natarajasana (Dancer Pose)

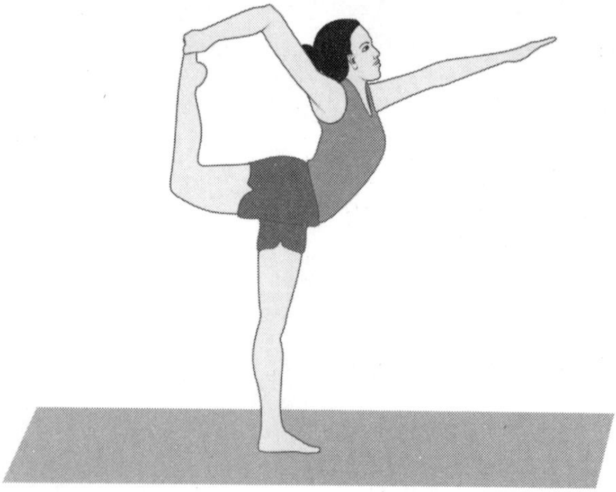

This is a very traditional posture that typifies one of the beautiful forms of the tandav nrittya (energetic dance) of Lord Shiva. Hence it is known as Nataraja (Lord Shiva's) pose.

Steps

a) Stand erect in tadasana (mountain pose).
b) Fix the drishti (gaze) on a spot in front of you.
c) Raise your left arm above your head with palms facing the front. With the right hand pick up the right leg and hold your feet.
d) Steady yourself here and feel centred.
e) Take a deep inhalation, and as you exhale, slowly bend forward and arch your back. Keep the spine straight. Simultaneously raise your right leg but maintain the balance on your left foot. Keep lifting the right leg till such time that the right thigh disappears from the frontal vision. The left arm will extend forward at an angle as shown in the illustration.

   Take a few breaths, let go slowly on an exhale and come back to tadasana (mountain pose) and relax.

   Repeat on the other side.

Benefits

This is a beautiful balancing posture that strengthens the legs, particularly the quadriceps, inner thighs and hamstrings, and improves concentration immensely. This posture also stretches the frontal upper body, opens up the chest and the vertebrae and strengthens the backbone.

17. Vrikṣasana (Tree Pose)

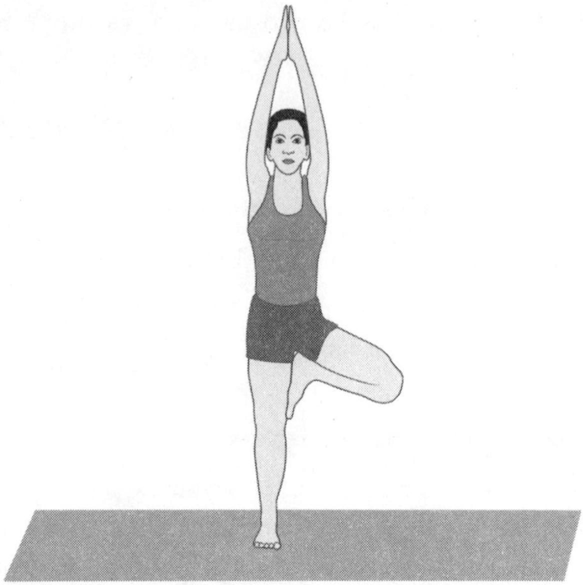

This asana is meditative and an excellent balancing posture.

Steps

a) Stand in tadasana (mountain pose) and take a deep inhalation, bend your left leg and rest it high on your right inner thigh near the joints.

b) Bring your hand to the prayer position first and fix your gaze or, if you can, close your eyes. Exhale.

c) Take another deep inhalation and, in the same prayer position, raise your arms upwards above your head, on an exhale.

Meditate and breathe. Release and repeat with the other leg.

Benefits

This posture has similar benefits as tadasana (mountain pose). But balancing on one leg makes it slightly more challenging than tadasana (mountain pose). This asana (posture) also improves balance, stability, concentration, grace and poise.

18. Ardha Chandrasana (Half-moon Pose)

(a)

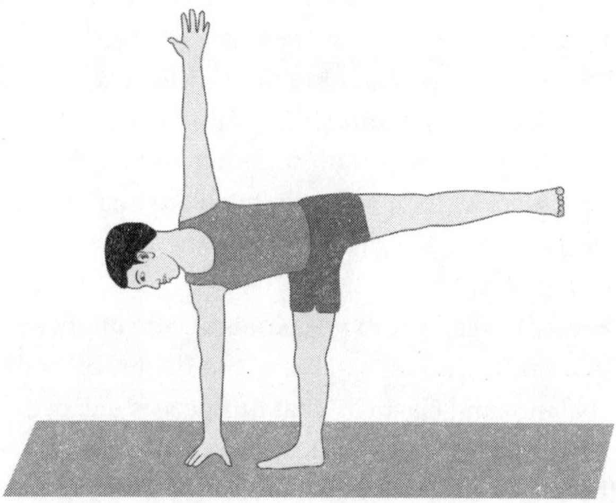

(b)

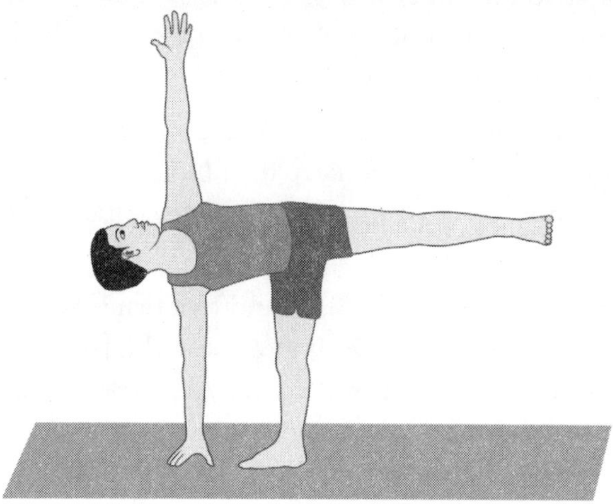

This is a balancing posture with a twist and you might want to use a prop (a wooden block) initially. Stretch, twist and balance is what this asana (posture) is all about.

Steps

a) From tadasana (mountain pose), follow the steps and come to virabhadrasana 3 (warrior pose 3) directly, because the half-moon pose is easier to achieve this way, sequentially.
b) Take a deep breath and shift your drishti (gaze) to a spot on the floor and as you do so, bring your right hand to the floor. Use a block for support if you are unable to reach the floor. Raise the left arm towards the ceiling. Exhale and keep breathing normally.
c) Take care to keep your knees straight. You might be tempted to bend it, as you aim to reach the floor. This will disturb the balance and elasticity that this pose is meant to achieve.
d) Practise till this stage until you are ready to take the stance fully. It is better to try this asana (posture) in increments and not push yourself.
e) When you are at ease in this position, take a deep breath and twist from your waist and turn the upper body to face the front on an exhale.
f) Look up and focus your gaze on the left hand. Do not strain your neck muscles and keep breathing.

   In this stance, your hip opens up together with the entire upper torso and you balance solely on your fingertips and right leg, with knee straight and foot firmly rooted on the floor. You will feel a deep stretch on the left side of your waist and alongside. As your body is able to bend more, you will be able to do away with the prop and bring your right hand all the way down to touch the floor.

   Take a deep breath and gently release the position on an exhale by bringing your foot down. Place both hands on your knees, look down and take a few breaths.

Repeat on the other side. Release the posture, come to tadasana (mountain pose) and relax.

Benefits

It is a great balancing posture and a hip, pelvic and chest opener. It tones the entire body and improves stability, concentration and elasticity of the body. It immensely puts to test the strength of your leg muscles and its ability to take the weight of your entire body.

19. Vasisthanasana (Side Plank Pose)

(a)

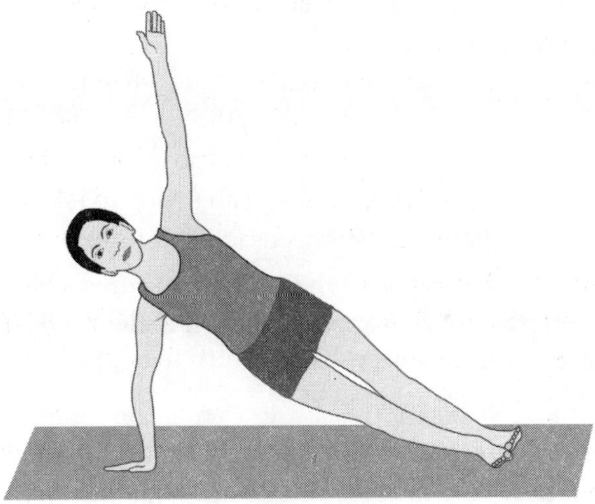

(b)

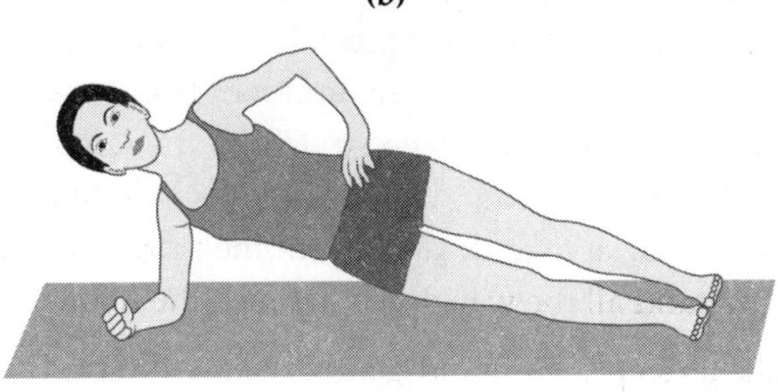

The side plank pose is a powerful asana (posture) and a complete body workout.

Steps

a) Come down on your hands and knees and get into the four-limbed high plank pose, as described in the surya namaskar (sun salutation) sequence.

b) Take a deep breath and as you exhale, twist your entire body to the right side, with the weight of your body evenly distributed on arms and core muscles. In this position the rim of your right foot should rest on the floor and the left foot will automatically take its position and graze your right foot.

c) As shown in illustration (a) apart from your hand and the rim of your foot, the entire body is suspended from the floor.

   If you find this too intense, you can rest on your forearm as shown in illustration (b).

   The adventurous ones, who want to take this a bit further, can lift their left leg parallel to the floor and further challenge their balance.

   Take a deep breath, release gracefully on an exhale and come to four-limbed high plank pose. Take a few breaths and repeat on the other side in the same manner. Finally release the posture and from high plank pose slowly lower your body to the floor and relax in savasana (corpse pose).

Benefits

This asana (posture) is a complete body workout and strengthens the wrists, biceps, triceps, quadriceps and immensely challenges your core strength. It is quite an intense balancing pose but not too hard to attain, once you have perfected the technique.

20. Garudasana (Eagle pose)

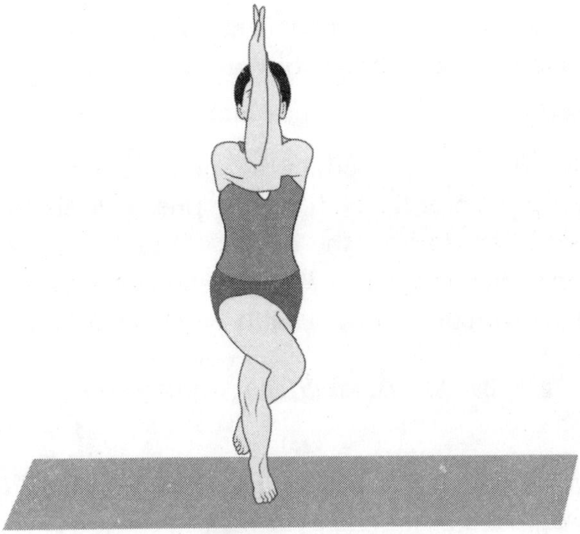

This asana (posture) is a bit tricky as you need to balance on one leg and also synchronise your hands and breathe. It is a beautiful stance to add that extra zest to your balancing series.

Steps

a) Start with tadasana (mountain pose) and get into utkatasana, the imaginary chair pose as explained earlier.

b) Now entwine your hands by placing the right arm over your left and try to press your palms as in anjali (prayer position). Because of the way your arms are entwined, there will be a slight misalignment in anjali, which is okay. Just the way it ought to be.

c) Now comes the tricky part. Focus on your drishti (gaze) and without losing your balance take a deep inhalation and on an exhale slowly place the back of your right thigh on the frontal left thigh and entwine it all the way to rest the right foot on your left calf.

d) Control the urge to stand up and remain seated. Keep breathing. On an exhale release the position gracefully without losing balance. Repeat with the other leg and reverse the arms position.

Benefits

This asana (posture) is good for the spine, shoulder joints and the lower portion of the body as it improves flexibility of the muscles and strengthens the thighs, calves and hips. It also helps concentration and memory as it stimulates the mind and body along with promoting stability and body balance.

21. Sirsasana (Head Stand Pose)

(a)

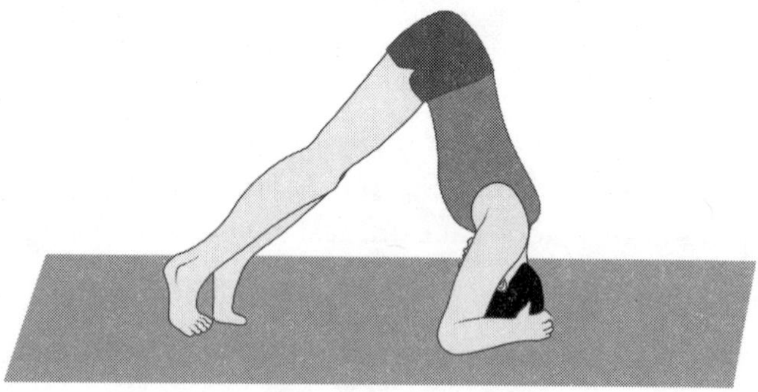

(b)

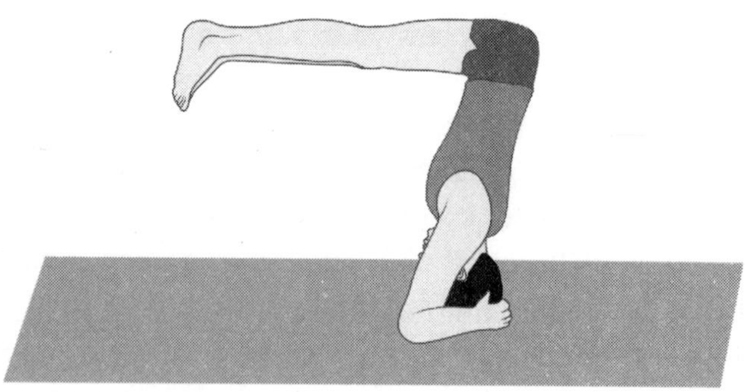

(c)

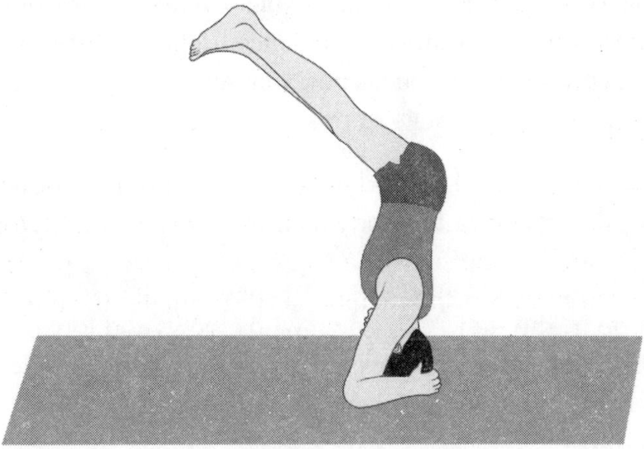

(d)

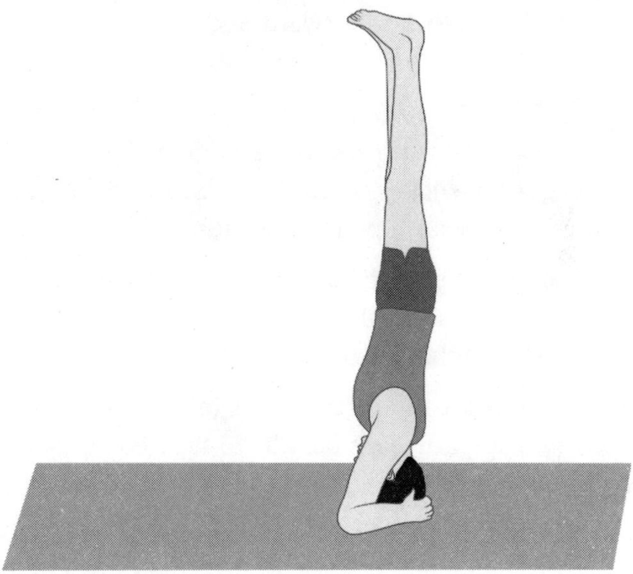

This is known as the king of all asana (postures). Sirsasana (Head stand pose) has similar benefits as sarvangasana (shoulder stand pose), the queen of all asana (postures).

Sirsasana (head stand pose) is best done under proper guidance as this is an extremely invigorating inversion posture. This asana (posture) is supposed to remove all ailments, cleanse your central nervous system and slow down the biological clock. Most people believe this to be an anti-ageing asana (posture).

Steps

a) Place a few blankets on the floor against the wall, to support the stance. Sit down with elbows and forearms on the blanket and clasp the fingers of both hands in order to rest the crown of your head on the palms.

b) Focus inward. Use wall support initially. Stand in an inverted V position, somewhat similar to the dolphin pose.

c) Slowly bring both legs forward and closer. Keep leaning towards the wall until you feel your spine straighten up against the wall.

d) Now slowly lift one leg and bring it down. Try this with the other leg. This will help to ease your back and get ready for the asana (posture), a preparatory step.

   (More seasoned practitioners just do it all at one go and in the centre of the room. But to get there, you need to follow these steps and that too under supervision).

e) When you feel ready lift both legs in a folded position or you may extend the legs parallel to the floor, as shown in the illustration (b).

   If you are not ready or feel that you may lose your balance, please do not stretch the legs. It is okay to bend them for balance. You are a yogi not an acrobat.

   Then slowly raise the legs up very gently as depicted in (c) and extend them upwards as illustrated in (d).

Release the position immediately. Once you have grasped the technique, and gained confidence, you can hold this stance, but until then please do not hurt yourself by being overambitious. Extreme care must be taken to not exert pressure on your neck.

Benefits

This posture improves the blood circulation in the entire body, concentration and memory, keeps the body supple, reduces stress by calming the mind, removes energy blockages and is good for the central nervous system. It strengthens the arms, neck, shoulders and backbone. It also develops core strength and relieves the legs of any pressure or pain. Chances of dementia, nervous disorders and diseases are said to considerably reduce if this asana (posture) is done daily with passion, patience and care. These benefits also apply to sarvangasana (shoulder stand pose).

Readers,

I have tried to simplify and explain the manner of achieving every asana (posture) in a logical manner, based on my learning and practice. I wish to conclude this part with a few general tips:

In any of the balancing series, if you happen to lose or falter in your stance, come back to the posture again but do not give up. This is what training the body is all about. Eventually your body will obey you and the mind will become the master of your body.

No matter what level of practice you may be at, even if you are able to comfortably attain the basic postures with props, you will be rewarded with the benefits. Hence please do not fret or struggle and allow time to show you the way.

Breathing pattern, focus on breath and engaging/ locking the bandhas (interior body locks) should become part and parcel of your yoga practice.

Part 3 – Daily Yoga Practice

(Seven-day regimen from my yoga journal)

17

Yoganomics

I would like to share with you a few words of wisdom of my various instructors which are noteworthy.

- No effort no gain – This is the basic principle of any discipline and yoga. One has to make an effort in order reap the rewards.
- Do not worry about pins and needles; it is just your nerves talking to you – Many of us start worrying and fidgeting when we experience pins and needles as we sit in a particular posture or when we meditate. This can be tolerated and its occurrence will reduce with practice. All you need to do is wiggle your legs and rub the toes to improve blood circulation and then resume your stance.
- Release the posture when you feel pain – Yoga is not about enduring pain. When you experience pain, something more than pins and needles or a painful discomfort, release the posture immediately and come to balasana (child's pose) to avoid sustaining an injury.
- Stay with your breath – This is one of the most important aspects in yoga practice. When the mind wanders bring back your attention by telling yourself:

"I know I am breathing in, as you inhale."

"I know I am breathing out, as you exhale."

- Triple pearls – Adho mukha svanasana (downward facing dog pose), malasana (garland pose) and setu bandhasana (bridge pose) serve well as the triple pearls of yoga. There will be days when you are unable to devote time for an hour long yoga practice or make it to the class. During such times, practise these three asana (postures) along with six rounds of surya namaskar (sun salutation) for a complete workout.

- Garlic or tonic of yoga – Adho mukha svanasana (downward facing dog pose) is known to be the garlic or tonic of yoga, as this is one of the easier inversion postures. It not only stretches and rejuvenates your body but also improves stamina and enables to engage the three bandhas (interior body locks) effortlessly.

Remember yoga is a dance – practise it with grace, poise and fervour.

18

Monday Regimen

Monday – This day of the week is usually the busiest, for most of us, particularly after a relaxed weekend. A perfect fit is yin practice to relieve stiffness of the body in a soothing manner.

a) Lie down in balasana (child's pose). With a deep inhalation extend further from your hips and open up the shoulders and keep stretching the arms forward. Try to lift your elbows off the floor with fingertips on the mat, inch a little forward and feel the stretch of your upper body. Be still and focus on the breath. Feel the body responding and relaxing. Think of nothing but your breath. Enjoy the peace within. Breathe normally.

b) Take a deep inhalation and, as you exhale, slowly come up on your hands and knees, known as the table top position and get ready for the cat and cow movements. Inhale as you arch your back as a cat. Exhale and round your back sucking in your abdomen inwards like a cow. Repeat this movement for a few times and try to draw number 8 by moving your body sideways, on either side. Remember to breathe steadily in ujjayi (oceanic) breaths.

c) Come back to table top position. With a deep inhalation draw your body backwards so as to rest your buttocks on the heels. With a deep exhalation energetically sink into adho mukha svanasana (downward facing dog pose). Adjust your body and keep cycling your legs till you feel comfortable in this asana (posture). Take a few breaths here.

d) Take a deep breath and extend your right leg backwards, as in downward facing dog with leg raise, and keep your left leg firm on the floor. On an exhalation, bring your right foot forward by bending your knee. Place your knee close to your little finger on the right hand with foot facing the left side. Gently lower yourself down. Prop up a cushion under the right buttock, if necessary. Your left leg ought to be firm, straight and extended backwards positioned along the centre of your mat. Keep your back and spine erect and stay in this pigeon pose. You should feel a deep stretch in the inner thigh, upper back and spine. In this position your upper body will lengthen from the hips and sit bones to stay rooted on the floor or cushion. Keep eyes closed and breathe gently. Focus on your breath. Stay here for two minutes.

e) Take another deep inhalation and slowly come all the way down to sleeping swan pose as you exhale. Rest forehead on a cushion or your forearm. If you feel too comfortable in this posture, try extending your arms forward and rest your forehead on the floor. Take a few breaths here. Stay still with eyes closed for another two minutes. Release and come back to pigeon pose with a deep inhalation and exhale as you once again sink into adho mukha svanasana (downward facing dog pose). Repeat the pigeon and sleeping swan pose on the other side.

f) From adho mukha svanasana (downward facing dog pose), slowly toggle your feet to the front of the mat and stay in uttanasana (forward bend pose) for a couple of breaths. Sway your body from side to side and release any tension in your hips, neck and shoulder joints. Feel light and wobbly like a rag doll.

g) Take a deep inhalation and bring your feet slightly more than hip-width apart. With a deep exhalation, sink into malasana (garland pose). Rest your forehead on the finger tips as your hands are in anjali (prayer position) and close your eyes and breathe. Stay still and meditate. Now the body is geared for a backbend.

h) Release the garland pose and lie down on your belly for the sphinx and seal pose. Get into the sphinx pose, close your eyes and lie still. Breathe and try to engage your mula bandha (root lock) without tightening the gluteus. Stay here for three minutes and relax. Take a deep breath and intensify the backbend into the seal pose, hold on for a minute and breathe normally. Take a deep inhalation, release and come back to sphinx pose and with a deep exhalation come all the way down to lie on your belly with head tilted to one side. Enjoy the relaxation of your muscles after the intensity of the backbend.

i) Now it is time for a forward bend to soothe your back. Raise your body and come to balasana (child's pose) and relax for a minute before getting ready for the next asana (posture).

j) Sit down in dandasana (staff pose) with the back and spine erect and if necessary place a tiny cushion under your sit bones. Bend and draw both legs towards yourself and come to baddha konasana (cobbler or butterfly pose). Once you are well adjusted in the pose, take a deep inhalation and come forward as you exhale. Do this in increments. Take another deep inhalation, exhale and bend a bit more until you are able to come down on the floor as much as possible. When your body reaches the level of resistance, do not push farther; instead, close your eyes, relax and breathe. Stay still and observe your breath.

   The yin practice ends here.

k) Release and get ready for the final pose which is ustrasana (camel pose). Perform this posture with care and caution by supporting your lower back and spine with both hands. Please remember to follow the steps as explained in Part 2 of the book. You must not hold this asana (posture). Repeat it one more time if you feel any tightness after the forward bend.

Tip

In case you feel tightness in your hips, you can also try the dragon pose or the frog pose which are great hip openers.

Finally relax in savasana (corpse pose). Stay here for ten to twelve minutes and breathe softly. Turn over to your side and sit up when ready.

Please note that in all yin postures as you inhale, lengthen a few millimetres, stretch and then relax. Take the postures in increments. It serves well to keep your eyes closed during yin yoga sessions. All yin postures are meant to be held for at least three minutes. Unsupported stance is not advisable and use of props during yin yoga sessions is highly recommended. It is good to not introduce too many asana (postures) in yin practice, as the focus is more on opening up the body, relaxation and melting in the moment.

19

Tuesday Regimen

It is good to start the Tuesday yoga practice with surya namaskar (sun salutation) series and follow it up with a few asana (postures) as stated below.

a) Lie down in savasana (corpse pose)and enjoy the relaxation process by focussing your breath and attention on the body, starting from your toes till the crown of your head. Relax and mindfully engage the bandhas (interior body locks). Lie still and resist the temptation to fidget. Feel the calmness permeate through your mind. Extend both arms above your head, take a deep breath and flex your toes inwards, as you stretch and elongate your body. Exhale and relax the toes. Repeat this again with toes flexed outwards.

b) Start with balasana (child's pose). Focus on your breath and keep eyes closed. Loosen your shoulder joints by tucking in your right arm below your chest and extending it towards the left side. After a few seconds, repeat this with your left arm towards the right side. The arm twist will loosen the shoulder joints and make it flexible.

c) Start the cat and cow movements. Move sideways from your hips and draw number 8, in clockwise and anticlockwise direction.

d) Take a deep inhalation, draw your body inwards and momentarily rest your buttocks on your heels and come to adho mukha svanasana (downward facing dog pose) with a deep exhalation. Take a few breaths here and enjoy the good stretch to your spine and back. Cycle your legs to loosen up the body.

e) With both feet firm on the floor, inch your upper torso backwards and hold both elbows with opposite hands, the crown of your head being just above the floor. If you have tight hamstrings, you may bend your knees slightly. Let your upper body hang loose like a rag doll. Relax your neck and facial muscles. Feel the blush on your cheeks. Sway from side to side.

f) Come up slowly and start with tadasana (mountain pose) and get ready to start the surya namaskar (sun salutation) series. Follow the stepwise sequence, as explained in Part 2, and repeat the series at least six times. Gradually increase it to ten rounds. Your body will begin to feel energised. Relax in savasana (corpse pose) for few seconds. Draw the legs to the chest and embrace with both arms, rock your body and sit up. With another robust movement, stand up and get ready to start the asana (posture).

g) With a swift jump, extend both legs sideways for utthita parsvakonasana (extended side angle pose). Start on your right side and feel the stretch alongside your left waist, hips, arms from shoulder onwards and the left leg. Stretch to the fullest and repeat in the same manner on the other side.

h) From utthita parsvakonasana (extended side angle pose), take it further to parivrtta parsvakonasana (revolved side angle pose). This is a perfect moment for the extra twist and turn, as the upper body is well-stretched and has become quite flexible after utthita parsvakonasana (extended side angle pose). Repeat on both sides. Come back to tadasana (mountain pose) for a few seconds.

i) It is time for a sideways bend with trikonasana (triangle pose). Use a prop and do not overstretch yourself. Be reasonable with your body and allow it to get flexible rather than forcing upon yourself. Repeat on both sides.

j) Parivrtta trikonasana (revolved triangle pose) is the next posture as the joints are well lubricated and you will find it easier to twist and turn. Repeat on both sides.

k) After the sideways bends and twists, it will be soothing to go for an intense forward bend and an inversion posture, prasarita padottanasana (wide legged forward bend pose) to energise and feel refreshed.

l) Come back to tadasana (mountain pose) for a few seconds and get ready for the seated asana (postures) after the power packed standing series.

m) Sit down in vajrasana (thunderbolt pose) to stimulate your mind and relax the body.

n) Extend legs forward and start with paschimottanasana (seated forward bend pose). Enjoy here for a few seconds with eyes closed and focus fully on your breath. Release and get ready for an intense backbend.

o) Ustrasana (camel pose) will be the last posture for the day and you may repeat this twice one after the other, but with slow and assured movements.

   Release and come to balasana (child's pose) to soothe your back. Stay in this posture for a few seconds.

p) Sit in gomukhasana (cow face pose) and start your eye exercises. Then rub both palms and cup your eyes for a few seconds. You will find a sense of calm descend over you.

q) Settle down in savasana (corpse pose). When you come out of this pose at the end of every session, you should turn over to one side and then rise slowly.

   It is sufficient to attain these asana (postures) to the

maximum that your body permits, hold for a few seconds and move on. Follow the steps and the breathing technique explained in Part 2 and remember to engage the body locks.

20

Wednesday Regimen

It is good to add momentum and agility during the midweek practice. Keeping this in mind, I have included postures which can be done in vinyasa style. The postures are the same but this style is more energetic since the sequences are done with continuous breathing pattern and every movement of the body is synchronised with your breath.

In vinyasa yoga practice, you are free to adjust the pace in accordance with your body stamina. It does not have to be too fast paced that it should make you breathless.

Begin with the warm up sequence as per Tuesday's regimen, starting with savasana (corpse pose) followed by balasana (child's pose) and the cat and cow movements.

A) Begin the surya namaskar (sun salutation) series with vinyasa breaths.

a) Stand in tadasana (mountain pose) or samasthiti. Take a few deep breaths here.

b) Take a deep inhalation and move to urdhva hastasana (raised hands pose).

c) Exhale and come down to uttanasana (forward bend pose).

d) Inhale to halfway lunge, the intermediary pose, extending the right leg backwards and quickly get to the four-limbed high plank pose.

e) Deeply exhale to chaturanga dandasana (four-limbed staff pose) and then come all the way down on the floor.

f) Inhale and move on to urdhva mukha svanasana (upward-facing dog pose).

g) Exhale and come to adho mukha svanasana (downward-facing dog pose).

h) Inhale and come down to halfway lunge, the intermediary pose, with right leg forward.

i) Exhale to uttanasana (forward bend pose).

j) Inhale and take the intense backbend pose.

k) Exhale and come back to tadasana (mountain pose).

l) As you repeat the above sequence synchronising your breath with every movement, it will get more intense and energising. Six rounds will fully prepare you for the next set of standing series. Take a few breaths in tadasana (mountain pose).

B) Standing Postures

a) With a deep inhalation raise arms above your head and come to urdhva hastasana (raised hands pose).

b) Exhale and sit in utkatasana (chair pose).

c) Deeply inhale and bring your palms to the heart's centre in anjali (prayer position) and extend your upper torso forward. Keep the spine erect. Stay in the seated position.

d) Exhale and twist to your left in parivrtta utkatasana (twisted chair pose). The right elbow should rest on the left thigh or above the knee. Whilst doing so, remember to engage your uddiyana bandha (abdominal lock). Twist your upper torso from the waist and look up. Please ensure that you do not rest your torso on your left thigh, it should twist and there ought to be a gap between your thigh and torso.

e) Take a deep inhalation and, upon an exhalation come back to utkatasana (chair pose). Another deep inhalation and, on an exhalation, take parivrtta utkatasana (twisted chair pose) to your right, in the same manner as described above. Take a deep inhale and on an exhale come back to utkatasana (chair pose) and then stand up in tadasana (mountain pose). Keep breathing.

f) Repeat the above set from utkatasana (chair pose) to parivritta utkatasana (twisted chair pose) one more time if you desire.

g) From tadasana (mountain pose) take a deep breath and on an exhale bend forward in uttanasana (forward bend pose). Inhale and lift half way with both hands resting on your knees and upper torso extended forwards. This is to prepare for the next move. Exhale and jump to four-limbed high plank pose. Inhale and on an exhalation, come down to chaturanga dandasana (four-limbed staff pose) first and then all the way down. Inhale into bhujangasana (cobra pose) or urdhva mukha svanasana (upward facing dog pose). Exhale and come to adho mukha svanasana (downward facing dog pose).

h) Take a few breaths here.

i) With a deep inhalation come to virabhadrasana 1 (warrior pose 1). Exhale and come to virabhadrasana 2 (warrior pose 2).

j) Position your legs for trikonasana (triangle pose). Inhale and take a deep exhale whilst bending sideways to your right. Open up shoulders and raise the left arm upwards. Simultaneously bring your right arm to hold the ankle or touch the floor, depending on the extent you can bend. Please do not force yourself. Inhale. Exhale and come up to the centre. Inhale. Exhale and take trikonasana (triangle pose) on your left side, in the manner described above. Inhale. Exhale and come to the centre position with both legs extended sideways. Take a deep inhale.

k) Exhale and bend forward in prasarita paddottanasana (wide legged forward bend pose).

l) Breathe softly and relax in this inversion posture and close your eyes. When you are ready, take a deep breath and on an exhale come back to tadasana (mountain pose).

m) Relax and get ready for the balancing postures with normal, regulated breathing pattern.

Vinyasa Practice ends here.

C) Balancing postures

a) Begin with natarajasana (dancer pose). Balance on your left leg and raise your left arm above the head. Bend right knee and hold the foot firmly with the right hand. Slowly as you exhale start kicking the right leg backwards and simultaneously bring your torso forward along with the left arm. Gradually the right thigh will be parallel to the floor. Release slowly and repeat on the other side.

b) Move onto virabhadrasana 3 (warrior pose 3). Keep your left foot rooted on the floor and swing the right leg forward and backwards, two-to-three times. Then slowly bring the leg behind and extend your torso forward with both arms stretched forward and raise the right leg as straight as possible, almost parallel to the floor. Balance in warrior pose 3. Freeze your drishti (gaze) at a spot on the floor and be steady. Repeat on the other side.

c) Next in sequence is ardha chandrasana (half-moon pose). Keep up the balance, bend down and place both hands or finger tips on either side of the left foot and steady yourself for the half-moon pose. Thereafter lift the right arm upwards and look up if you can. Repeat on the other side.

d) Vriksasana (tree pose) is the last of the balancing series. Repeat on both sides.

It is always nice to end the practice with a few prone poses to strengthen the back.

D) Prone Postures

a) Lie down on the stomach and toggle both feet together with chin or forehead on the floor for bhujangasana (cobra pose). Rotate your shoulders and release any built-up tension in shoulder joints. Press both palms on the floor and take a deep inhale as you rise up, hold and then exhale as you come down. Repeat this one more time.

b) Get ready for salabhasana (locust pose). Place both palms on the floor, facing inwards, under your thighs for elevation. Inhale and raise right leg without bending the knees. Exhale and bring it down. Now repeat with the other leg. Finally with a deep inhale raise both legs and hold for a few seconds. On an exhalation bring both legs down.

c) Take a deep inhalation as you raise yourself and exhale into balasana (child's pose).

d) Turn around for ananda balasana (happy baby pose) and enjoy.

e) Relax completely in savasana (corpse pose).

A pat on the back is well deserved after this vigorous vinyasa session!

21

Thursday Regimen

After a powerful vinyasa practice, it is time to sublimate Thursday with a perfect blend of meditation and breathing exercises (basic diaphragm breathing only) before starting the warm up movements and asana (postures).

Begin by sitting in a comfortable cross legged position. If necessary you could use a cushion to support the sit bones. Tilt the head slightly downward so that your chin is not held high and rest your tongue lightly on the upper jaw. Place both hands on the knee or lock them and place it just below your navel.

Once you are comfortable, close your eyes and take a few soft yet long breaths. Then slowly move onto ujjayi (oceanic) breaths. Focus on your breath and take a deep inhalation, fill your lungs with pure air and then allow the air to fill your belly. Feel your belly expand. For instance, if you take six seconds to inhale; pause for two to three seconds and then slowly exhale the air fully from your lungs and belly and feel the contraction. The exhalation should be longer than your inhalation, ideally for twelve seconds, but if you can manage eight-to-ten seconds, it is considered to be a good start. As you exhale, your diaphragm will contract. Try to feel the contraction and lock the uddiyana bandha (abdominal lock). Remember to lock your mula bandha (root lock) throughout the breathing exercise.

Repeat this inhale-pause-exhale, a few times, say approximately ten times (not more) because by then you will feel very relaxed and centred. Finally take a deep breath and chant OM by mouthing Aaa...Ooo...Mmm.... You should feel the buzz in your ears as you do so. Rub both palms, cup them and place over your eyes and the rest of the body. Slowly open your eyes.

a) Come to baddha konasana (cobbler or butterfly pose) and feel the stretch in your inner thighs. Press your knees to the floor. Hold your toes together and look ahead. Cradle your right leg and hold it on one side, as if rocking a baby.

   Repeat on the other side with the left leg. Remember to breathe.

b) Now stretch the legs forward and wiggle it like a wiper. Widen the legs apart till you feel the stretch in your inner thighs. You might want a prop under the sit bones, so as to keep your spine straight. Inhale deeply and raise both arms above the head. Exhale and bend all the way down to hold the left toes. Inhale as you come up and exhale to reach out on the other side to hold the right toes with both hands. Repeat this for a few times.

c) Slowly bring your legs together and take a deep breath. As you exhale, move on to paschimottanasana (seated forward bend pose). Hold the feet or toes and let your crown rest on the farthest part of the leg.

d) Come down on your hands and knees and start the cat and cow movements to exercise your spine and back.

e) Take an intense backbend with ustrasana (camel pose). Exhale as you release the posture.

f) Relax for a few seconds in balasana (child's pose).

g) Slowly rise up to tadasana (mountain pose) and sink into this posture for a few seconds. Feel grounded and freeze your drishti (gaze).

h) After the above warm up, you will feel energised for the surya namaskar (sun salutation) in vinyasa style, as explained in the Wednesday regimen, moving with every breath and being mindful of your movements. Repeat for six to ten rounds. Relax in savasana (corpse pose).

i) Take a deep inhalation and come to naukasana (boat pose) as you exhale. Breathe and fix your drishti (gaze) and hold on for a few seconds or as long as you can.

j) Release the posture and lie down in savasana (corpse pose). Immediately come back to naukasana (boat pose) one more time and relax in to savasana (corpse pose).

k) Take a deep inhalation and move on to setu bandhasana (bridge pose) as you exhale. Hold on for a minute. Release slowly to savasana (corpse pose). Repeat this one more time.

l) Take a deep inhalation and as you exhale raise your legs upwards at right angle to the body. Take another deep inhalation and as you exhale, extend both legs backwards to halasana (plow pose). Stay here with eyes closed for a minute and breathe. You will feel much energised as you lock the three bandhas (interior body locks).

m) With this renewed energy move on to sarvangasana (shoulder stand pose). Stay still and lock your bandhas (interior body locks). Breathe. Release the posture, slowly on an exhale and come all the way down to savasana (corpse pose).

n) Take matsyasana (fish pose) as the next and final asana (posture) as a contra pose.

o) Come back to savasana (corpse pose) and relax completely.

22

Friday Regimen

Friday – This day of the week is good to focus on opening up your hips, connective tissues and tendons to bring renewed energy in your body. What better way than yin yoga for some more restorative postures?

a) Start with the warm up asana (postures) viz. balasana (child's pose), cat and cow movements and adho mukha svanasana (downward facing dog pose). Keep cycling your legs slowly in the downward facing dog pose and take a few breaths.

b) Inhale and raise your right leg as high as possible by keeping it straight. Then slowly bend the knee towards the right and open up your right hips. Your right foot should be visible from under the armpit of your left arm. Exhale and bring the right foot down. In the same manner repeat with the left foot to open up your left hips.

c) Toggle both feet together and bring your bent upper torso close to the legs and hold your big toe. Stay still in this inversion pose of padangushtasana (forward bend and toe hold pose) for two minutes. Feel the blood rush to your face, relax your facial muscles and keep breathing.

d) Take a deep inhalation and sit down in malasana (garland pose) as you exhale. Continue to breathe and relax. Stay here for a couple of minutes.

e) Release the posture, sit down and stretch both legs forward. Wiggle your legs like a wiper and then get ready for the shoelace pose, a variation of gomukhasana (cow face pose).

Follow the steps as mentioned in Part 2 to settle down comfortably with a prop to support your back or sit bone for two minutes on both sides.

f) The next in the sequence is supta virasana (reclining hero pose). Take a deep inhalation and on an exhale as you lower yourself rest the elbows and support your back and spine with both hands. Slowly let the body melt in this asana (posture) for few minutes. Use the prop for back support. Close your eyes and breathe. Take a deep breath and release the position slowly on an exhale by supporting your back with both hands and rest on the elbows first before coming all the way up.

g) Sink into balasana (child's pose) to soothe your back.

h) Get ready for baddha konasana (butterfly or cobbler pose) for an intense forward bend. Remember to take the bend in increments and as far as you can. The important thing is to stay still and be able to hold this posture. Use a prop under both legs/knee for support.

i) Release and get ready for the therapeutic sphinx and seal pose to balance the effect of the above asana (posture). Relax in sphinx pose and then change over to seal pose and hold for a few seconds. Release and come back to sphinx pose and hold for a minute before coming all the way down to lie on your belly. Relax totally with head turned to one side, and arms alongside.

j) Move on to the dragon or frog pose for opening up your hips and joints.

k) The final posture will be viparita karani (legs up the wall pose) for massaging the tendons and ligaments. Close your eyes and relax for a while before concluding the session with savasana (corpse pose). Lie absolutely still for ten minutes with eyes closed and be mindful of your body being supported by the earth and feel the sensation in each and every part of your body. When you are ready to get up, slowly turn onto one side and sit up.

23

Saturday Regimen

As the week draws to a close, it would be ideal to go through a blend of asana (postures) for body balance and strength. In any of the balancing postures, if you feel you are losing your balance, do not give up and come back to the asana (posture) with more determination.

Follow the pattern of starting with savasana (corpse pose), balasana (child's pose) and the cat and cow movements similar to the Tuesday regimen and start the surya namaskar (sun salutations) for six to ten rounds. Relax in savasana (corpse pose) for a few breaths.

The new series starts now:

a) Turn on to your right side and start with anantasana (lying sideways and leg lift pose) for a nice stretch alongside the waist, hips and inner thighs. Bring this asana (posture) on with a smile. The challenge is to balance your entire body weight on one side without swaying. Repeat on the other side. Release the posture and lie on your back.

b) Inhale deeply and as you exhale raise yourself to naukasana (boat pose). Breathe softly. Freeze your drishti (gaze) so that you are able to maintain balance and challenge your core strength.

c) Lie down in savasana (corpse pose) for two seconds. Inhale deeply and on an exhale take a back bend with setu bandhasana (bridge pose). If you wish to intensify it further move on to urdhva dhanurasana (wheel pose).

Keep breathing.

d) Gently release the above posture and come back to savasana (corpse pose) for a couple of breaths.

e) It will be ideal to move on to halasana (plow pose) and lock your bandhas (interior body locks) in this posture to direct the flow of energy within the body.

f) Sit up and get ready for two sets of ustrasana (camel pose) for the extreme back bend as a contra posture to halasana (plow pose).

g) Release and come back to savasana (corpse pose) for a minute or two.

h) Your body is now more flexible and hence move on to sarvangasana (shoulder stand pose). Even then remember to take it in increments. Close your eyes and stay in this asana (posture) for a minute or two or longer, if you can. Please do not force yourself. Your body should automatically let you stay. Lock your bandhas (interior body locks).

i) Release slowly, step by step and come back to savasana (corpse pose). Take a few breaths here. Your body will feel very light at this stage, almost as if you are floating. This is a beautiful sensation that you need to cherish and enjoy.

j) Energise with matsyasana (fish pose) and get ready for a prone asana (posture) to strengthen your back.

k) Lie on your belly with arms alongside, fists clenched and forehead to the floor. As explained earlier, try the half locust pose first, by raising one leg at a time. Then raise both legs for the complete salabhasana (locust pose). Release and relax with head to one side.

l) Thereafter get ready for dhanurasana (bow pose). With forehead on the floor hold both ankles, take a deep inhalation and lift your torso and both legs off the floor.

Hold and breathe. Try to balance on your lower abdomen and thighs. The spine and back will curve finely increasing the suppleness. Release on an exhale and relax with head to one side.

Turn over and stand up for the final set of standing series.

m) Natarajasana (dancer pose) or garudasana (eagle pose) followed by vriksasana (tree pose) as explained in the Wednesday schedule will be a good fit to end this session with poise and grace.

n) Finally sit down in vajrasana (thunderbolt pose) or gomukhasana (cow face pose), depending on how your body feels and start eye rotation movements. This will help to reduce eye strain after a busy week.

o) Sit quietly in vajrasana (thunderbolt pose) for five minutes with eyes closed. Start your basic breathing exercise as explained in the Thursday regimen to feel calm and centred.

p) With this nice feeling, lie down as quietly as possible in savasana (corpse pose) and breathe softly. Fill your mind with positive thoughts and emotions, acknowledge in your mind all the good events of the week and consciously try and let go of anything negative.

q) Finally, thank the Lord for giving you the spirit, inclination and health for a daily yoga practice and feel blessed!

24

Sunday Regimen

The start of the week is the time to contemplate. I would recommend that this be your no exercise day and you devote half-an-hour for meditation and introspection. Needless to say, meditation should be part of your daily activity apart from yoga practice.

During the initial stage start with ten minutes of silence and stillness and this can be gradually increased to twenty minutes to half an hour. The challenge lies in being regular and disciplined and not letting go of your practice.

On this day of the week, you could also include basic pranayama (breathing technique) together with the technique of engaging the three bandhas (interior body locks).

I would like to conclude with a prayer to the Guru (teacher) and the all-pervading Eternal Power to bless all of us with purity of thought, deed and action so that we are able to spring out of bed, every day with childlike enthusiasm and face our life as if it is the first, last and the best.

> *Brahmanandam Parama Sukhadam*
> *Kevalam Jnana Murtim*
> *Dwanda Ateetam Gagana Sadrisham*
> *Tattwam Asyadi Lakshyam;*
> *Ekam Nityam Vimalam Achalam*
> *Sarvadee Sakshi Bhootham*
> *Bhava Ateetam Triguna Rahitam*
> *Sadgurum Tam Namami*

"I prostrate to my Guru and God, who is eternal bliss, giver of supreme happiness, who is absolute knowledge and beyond the pairs of opposites, vast like ether, who is attained through assertions like tat twam asi ('that thou art'). He is one, eternal, pure and changeless, witness of the mind, one who transcends all changes and modifications, devoid of the three modes of prakriti (nature)."

(Translation courtesy – The Divine Life Society, Sivananda Ashram, Rishikesh, Himalayas)

• • •

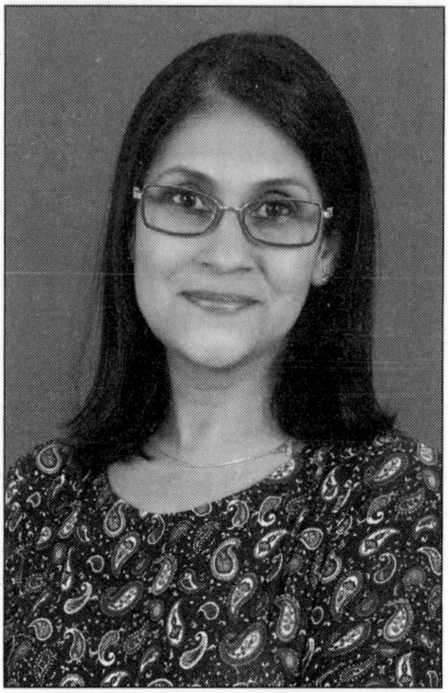

Revathi Raj Iyer is a freelance writer, book reviewer, company director, service volunteer and yoga/fitness enthusiast. She has worked in the corporate field for over a decade and bid adieu to a rewarding career with a multinational to become a full time mum. Bombay is her hometown and Baroda her abode after marriage. This was followed by a long stint in Fiji Islands, where she also started to learn yoga, pursued the training in New Zealand and continues her passion after moving to India. She lives in Ahmedabad.